5:2
VEGGIE
AND VEGAN

Also by the author:

The 5:2 Good Food Kitchen

5:2 Your Life

The Ultimate 5:2 Diet Recipe Book

The 5:2 Diet Book

The Boot Camp

Soul Fire

Old School Ties

Brown Owl's Guide to Life

The Self-Preservation Society

The Starter Marriage

The Secret Shopper series

5:2

VEGGIE
AND VEGAN

*DELICIOUS VEGETARIAN AND VEGAN
FASTING RECIPES TO HELP YOU
LOSE WEIGHT AND FEEL GREAT*

KATE HARRISON

First published in Great Britain in 2017
by Orion Publishing Group Ltd
Carmelite House, 50 Victoria Embankment,
London, EC4Y 0DZ

An Hachette UK Company

1 3 5 7 9 10 8 6 4 2

Text © Kate Harrison 2017

The right of Kate Harrison to be identified as the author
of this work has been asserted in accordance with
the Copyright, Designs and Patents Act 1988.

A CIP catalogue record for this book
is available from the British Library.

ISBN: 9781409171263

Photography: Faith Mason
Props: Clare Sivell and Emily Barrett
Food styling: Nicola Richman
Consultant dietician: Catherine Kidd

Printed and bound by CPI Group

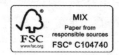

MIX
Paper from
responsible sources
FSC® C104740

Every effort has been made to ensure that the information in the book is accurate.
The information in this book may not be applicable in each individual case so it is advised
that professional medical advice is obtained for specific health matters and before
changing any medication or dosage. Neither the publisher nor author accepts any legal
responsibility for any personal injury or other damage or loss arising from the use of
the information in this book. In addition if you are concerned about your diet or
exercise regime and wish to change them, you should consult a health practitioner first.

Every effort has been made to fulfil requirements with regard to
reproducing copyright material. The author and publisher will be
glad to rectify any omissions at the earliest opportunity.

www.orionbooks.co.uk

Contents

PART 4: 5:2 RESOURCES   339

5:2 and veggie food

THE PERFECT MATCH FOR GOOD HEALTH AND STAYING IN SHAPE

May 2017

Dear reader,

Do you want to lose weight and enjoy delicious food that is packed with the nutrients your body needs to function at its best? Are you aiming to stay in good shape, have more energy and free yourself from yo-yo dieting? Then you're in the right place…

5:2 Veggie and Vegan combines two brilliant approaches to good health. **Intermittent fasting** is a proven, simple strategy to help you reach and maintain the right weight for you – and it also helps your body fight disease. **Plant-based eating** can reduce your risk of heart disease and cancer, lower your shopping bills and lessen your impact on the environment.

But the best bit? **Veggie and vegan food tastes fantastic**. The recipes in this book prove that you'll never miss out on flavour: from Indian breakfast pancakes, Sweet potato and chilli soup and Chestnut mushroom sausage rolls to Saucy miso aubergine, Veggie tikka masala, One-pot pea and white wine spaghetti and Margarita fruit salad, this lifestyle will keep your taste buds *very* happy. How do I know? Because it's how I eat. I've been a veggie for all my adult life, and I've been 5:2ing for five brilliant years.

How this book works

Part 1 explains the **basics of vegetarian and vegan nutrition**, the **principles of intermittent fasting** and how you can combine these approaches to be healthy and slim.

Part 2 is packed with over **80 delicious veggie and vegan recipes** that are all suitable for Fast Days and are so good you'll want to enjoy them on non-fasting days, too. All ingredients are individually **calorie-counted, to make them super-easy to adapt**.

If you need a little inspiration, alongside many of these recipes you'll find the real-life stories of people who've transformed their weight and health by combining 5:2 with veggie food.

Part 3 makes fasting days easy, with suggested **meal plans** and advice for non-fasting days. It also includes the

5:2 Know-how section, which is full of tips about savvy shopping, cooking shortcuts, batch-cooking ideas and stocking your 5:2 store cupboard, fridge and freezer.

Finally, **Part 4** has resources including a veggie food-focused **calorie counter** and suggestions for further reading about 5:2 and the veggie or vegan diet.

Why this book?

So why should you read on? Because veggie food and 5:2 are the perfect combination – and I'm living proof of that theory. I've been a veggie for three decades now, but despite my healthy diet I always struggled with my weight – until I started intermittent fasting.

I lost over two stone (31lb/14kg) in six months and, more importantly, I've kept the weight off now for five years. I still fast at least once a week for the health benefits: not just the extra energy and focus that it brings me, but also for the potential it offers to reduce my chances of developing type 2 diabetes, cancer and heart disease.

It's not just me, more than 55,000 people in the 5:2 Facebook group (facebook.com/groups/the52diet) are also sharing great results, and many of their experiences are included in this book. I set up the group with half a dozen others when I started experimenting with intermittent fasting in 2012, and now it has members from all over the world. And you can join us, too!

I'm not a professional chef, but I am a passionate home cook, and I love the challenge of making meat-free meals that also satisfy dedicated carnivores. I'm not a 'clean-eating' zealot, but I do love good food.

My background as an investigative journalist means that I am determined to get the answers to questions about health, weight loss and the food in our shops. Most of all, I believe in 5:2, and I want to share what I've learned.

Over to you

Discover how 5:2 combined with veggie food is about freedom, great food and feeling fantastic. And please get in touch to share *your* journey: join the Facebook group, visit the5-2dietbook.com – or you can say hi to me via Twitter @katewritesbooks.

Kate Harrison

Important safety note

You should always consult a doctor before making dietary changes.

This book is written for information only and is not intended as medical advice, or as a substitute for medical advice, diagnosis or treatment.

Children, teenagers, pregnant and breastfeeding women shouldn't fast.

If you have a chronic condition or diabetes, it's particularly important that you consult your doctor, specialist or diabetes nurse before embarking on 5:2 or any diet. Many people with type 2 diabetes or metabolic syndrome have had success with this way of eating, but it's essential that you do this under supervision, especially if you are taking medication.

If you have any history of eating disorders, you should also consult a doctor before making any dietary change, including 5:2.

Neither the author nor publisher or associates can be held responsible for any loss or claim resulting from the use or misuse of information and suggestions contained in this book, or for the failure to take medical advice.

Finally, never disregard professional medical advice or delay medical treatment because of something you have read in this book.

1

A GUIDE
TO THE VEGGIE
5:2
LIFE

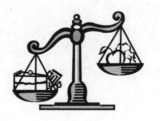

The good life

AN INTRODUCTION TO 5:2 VEGETARIAN AND VEGAN EATING

5:2 and veggie food is a match made in heaven: you get lots of food for your calories on a Fast Day and it's so nutritious, too.

KAREN, ENGLAND

We were doing 5:2 for over a year before we became vegan/vegetarian, and that made it very easy to change and adapt to our new lifestyle. We don't miss meat at all.

LIZ AND RAYMOND, AUSTRALIA

Veggie eating is definitely more creative, and people always comment about how good our food is, even on a Fast Day.

JO, SOUTH AFRICA

It's now nearly five years since intermittent fasting and 5:2 became the talk of the health and weight-loss world. In that time, hundreds of thousands of people have discovered that this way of life is sustainable, flexible and healthy.

In the same period, vegetarian and vegan lifestyles have been taking centre stage, as celebrities and scientists alike raise awareness of the health and environmental benefits of this way of eating. Many studies show a good veggie diet can reduce the risk of cancer or heart disease – and avoiding meat has less impact on the environment, as well as reducing animal suffering.

And it's not an all or nothing choice; many people aren't cutting out meat or fish entirely, but are simply choosing more plant-based options.

For me, fasting and veggie food work in perfect harmony. Too many 'trendy' diets are all about restrictions – whether it's the caveman 'rules' of a Paleo regime or the heavy bacon, steak and seafood plans of extreme low-carbing. Intermittent fasting, on the other hand, is flexible and easy – perfect for anyone who loves fresh and varied food. And, of course, most fresh vegetables are naturally low in calories and packed with flavour, so you can enjoy great meals even when you're cutting down for two days a week.

Let's look in more detail at the two approaches we're combining in this book: 5:2 fasting and plant-based eating.

What is 5:2?

5:2 is the most flexible approach to weight control and health you'll ever find.

On two days a week you cut your calorie consumption to around 25 per cent of what your body needs, and on the other five days, you eat normally.

It's sustainable

All weight-loss diets have the same basic logic: you must **consume less energy through food than you're using up in your everyday life**. The difference is how you achieve that 'calorie gap'.

Most diets expect you to deprive yourself every day. 5:2 is different because it concentrates the calorie-counting and restriction to just two days. Yes, your two 'fasting' day calorie limits are strict – **around 500 calories for women, 600 for men,** which are based on roughly a quarter of the daily average energy needs of 2000 calories per day for women, 2400 for men. But with a veggie or vegan diet you can stay within the Fast Day limit and still eat well.

On the other days of the week you're not having to calorie-count at every meal but are free to eat out, celebrate family occasions and enjoy the foods you love. The aim is simply to eat a balanced diet.

This approach means you're **more likely to sustain intermittent fasting long term than you are to keep one of the conventional weight-loss diets on offer.** Your social life won't be disrupted and you won't obsess over forbidden foods. Instead of restricting your food options, this way of eating empowers us to make good choices.

It's cheap

Weight loss isn't the whole story; **5:2 is also a cheaper** way to eat because you're consuming less, and unlike many weight-loss diets, you don't replace 'normal' food with expensive branded supplements or meal replacements.

It puts us back in touch with our body's signals

5:2 helps us **relearn what appetite feels like,** and to recognise the difference between eating to satisfy our appetite (a good response to our body's signals) and eating because we're bored, stressed, upset or thirsty (a case of crossed wires).

It has health benefits

Fasting also has potential health benefits, which are very motivating. Although this approach places your body under short-term stress, that stress is positive; it **encourages cell repair** and can help **protect against inflammation and damaging changes that cause ageing and disease**.

Finding a strategy for staying healthy in a world that promotes eating

Our prehistoric ancestors followed a 'fast/feast' pattern of eating; they took in as much energy as possible in the 'good' times, when plant foods were abundant or when hunters brought back an animal to cook, and focused on survival in leaner times, and their bodies adapted to cope and also to thrive.

Now, though, most of us can eat or snack whenever we wish: we're given the hard sell to make us want processed foods; and many of us actively avoid getting even slightly hungry. For the first time in history, excess weight is a bigger health threat worldwide than starvation: according to the World Health Organization, 65 per cent of the world's population now live in a country where obesity and weight gain kill more people than being underweight. That's at least 2.8 million people dying unnecessarily every year.

And with 39 per cent of the world's adults overweight and 13 per cent categorised as obese, it's not just the length of our lives that are affected, it's the quality, too, with chronic diseases related to obesity causing immeasurable suffering. Being overweight increases your risk of developing type 2 diabetes, cardiovascular disease as well as 13 types of cancer, including breast, bowel and kidney. Yet even though we know this, as individuals we often feel helpless about making the changes we know we should.

The reasons why weight is now such a problem are the subject of endless – and urgent – debate. Aside from the widespread availability of a vast range of processed foods, other pressures on us include:

- flawed advice on meal frequency and powerful marketing messages that suggest we should never allow ourselves to get even slightly hungry
- a natural survival instinct that makes us want to eat to build up fat reserves (for a famine that never actually comes)
- a reduction in knowledge about how to cook and food preparation

- less time to shop and prepare food at home
- our own personal responses – emotional and physical – to food.

It adds up to what researchers call an 'obesogenic' environment. With so many pressures on each of us, it's amazing that anyone manages to stay a healthy weight. Old-fashioned calorie-counting has worked for some people who want to lose weight, but many of us find resisting temptation all day, every day, is hard, if not impossible.

That's why 5:2 is different – it doesn't call for self-denial 24/7. Plus it encourages biological changes which can help our bodies to function better.

How can fasting help our bodies?

Going without food stresses the body – in a good way. Exercise is another example of positive stress or 'hormesis'. When you take an exercise class, go for a jog or lift some weights, you're putting your heart, lungs and muscles under stress, but your body responds by getting stronger and fitter. At first, it may feel uncomfortable because it's unfamiliar, but for healthy adults, fasting is safe (see page 39 for a reminder of who shouldn't fast). Contrary to the myths, short-term intermittent fasting, or planned meal-skipping, won't damage your metabolism or make you unwell. Instead, it helps in the following ways:

- **Improves insulin response:** Longer gaps between meals means insulin levels have chance to drop,

14

allowing us to burn body fat rather than store more for energy. Our blood sugar can thus fall to healthier levels and our body's response to insulin can also improve, reducing our chances of developing type 2 diabetes.

- **Short-term fasting can speed up metabolism,** the rate at which we use energy, which helps us lose weight or maintain a healthy weight. It has also been shown to help us have a better ratio of fat to muscle than conventional, everyday, very low-calorie diets.

- **Enables cell repair:** When they're not processing food, our bodies use the time to do 'housekeeping' at cellular level. In response to possible food shortages, the body carries out repairs to damaged cells (autophagy), or kills off those that can't be rescued (apoptosis). These processes may reduce the risk of cancers developing or growing.

- **May reduce damaging inflammation:** Studies on humans who undertake intermittent fasting have shown improvements in the biological 'markers' of future illness. These markers can predict the likelihood of developing cancer and cardiovascular disease. Inflammation in particular is associated with many diseases, including diabetes, heart disease, cancer, autoimmune conditions such as rheumatoid arthritis, and dementia. Some studies have shown that people who fast intermittently have lower levels of pro-inflammatory cytokines and CRP (C-reactive protein).

- **Boosts focus:** Concentration can be improved by short-term fasting, as certain proteins and hormones that influence focus, memory and mood are activated. On an evolutionary level, the smarter and more resourceful humans were in times of famine, the higher their chances of survival.

- **May reduce risk of degenerative conditions:** Longer-term fasting may protect the brain from ageing and reduce the chances of neurodegenerative conditions such as Alzheimer's disease and Parkinson's. Most of the research in this area so far has focused on animals, due to the difficulty of conducting human trials; and in studies involving mice and rats, fasting helped delay the onset and decrease symptoms in those genetically susceptible to degenerative brain conditions.
- **May improve life expectancy:** In some animal studies, a controlled, calorie-restricted diet has been shown to increase the length of time the animals stayed healthy *and*, in some cases, overall life expectancy. Of course, adult humans control what and when they eat, so it's harder to maintain a very low-calorie intake indefinitely. Intermittent fasting can be a more acceptable way to reduce energy consumption longer term.

This is an overview of the benefits, but for much more information about studies in humans and animals, and also a specific look at the effect of fasting on women's health, see the Further reading section on page 363, or my first book, *The 5:2 Diet Book*.

Why go veggie?

Ask 100 different vegetarians about their diet – and the reasons behind it – and you'll get 100 different answers.

I'm a vegan because it's such a small thing to do to improve the welfare and happiness of animals. Becoming vegan is no difficulty at all and the amount of misery it potentially stops is huge.

MARK

I have been veggie for three years, I work with dementia patients and I firmly believe that all the additives in our foods and meats contribute to this awful disease. Also I love animals and their welfare is uppermost in my mind.

SALLY

I'm veggie for the environment! It makes me feel really good every day to know how much water, land and resources I'm saving through my diet.

SUSAN

I grew up with animals...I loved the calves, pigs, ducks and rabbits and as a six-year-old I suddenly realised where the meat for the Sunday dinners came from, so I refused to eat my friends!

MIRA

I turned veggie when I was nine, 44 years ago, and have never eaten meat since. It wasn't that I was (or am) a great animal-lover, I just couldn't face putting flesh in my mouth, let alone chewing and swallowing it. I remember hearing an interview with a pop star who was asked what he would do if he saw bacon in the fridge. Wouldn't he want to eat it? 'No more than if I saw a brick in the fridge,' he replied.

KEVIN

To me, farming of livestock ultimately sees sentient life as a commodity and just a route to a product. There is no real value ascribed to that life itself – to freedom, happiness, longevity. When I realised it was possible to be vegan, I felt I had to try to live that way.

ALI

My father and his side of the family are all hunters so I was raised in an environment where hunting was the norm. I decided to go vegetarian on 14 January 2016 and, even though everyone told me it was just a phase, I'm still going strong. I can still eat healthy and delicious food without any other species having to die for me.

ISABELLE

My parents were both big meat eaters. My mum died of bowel cancer at 54, and on reading links between the two, I decided that no burger is worth that. We brought our kids up to make up their own minds; my daughter isn't a full veggie, my sons are. My youngest told us at eight he was never going to eat meat and even reads sweet wrappers to make sure they are animal product-free.

NINA

Concerns about **animal welfare, agricultural methods, the environment and our own health** are high on the list of reasons why people choose to follow a vegetarian or vegan diet. Here's a quick guide to the benefits of this way of eating, or for simply increasing the number of veg-based meals you eat…

Good health

Many studies have shown that a well-balanced vegetarian diet can reduce your risk of heart disease and cancer, and may help you live longer.

- Vegetarians have healthier BMI, cholesterol and blood sugar results, according to a 2016 review of almost 100 clinical studies by scientists in Florence. It reported significantly better results for blood sugar, BMI and cholesterol in vegetarians and vegans, compared to omnivores. The studies also showed that a vegetarian diet lowered the risk of coronary heart disease by 25 per cent and of all types of cancer by 8 per cent (15 per cent in the case of vegans).

- Major research in the US has focused on studying over 77,000 vegetarians and vegans who are members of the Seventh-day Adventist Church, which recommends a veggie diet, among other health measures. One of the studies, published in 2013, showed a 55 per cent lower risk of developing high blood pressure, a 25–49 per cent lower risk of type 2 diabetes, and a 23 per cent lower risk of bowel and other intestinal cancers. The results for heart disease were also positive, with between a 26 per cent and a 68 per cent lower risk of dying from heart disease and stroke, and a 48 per cent lower risk of dying from breast cancer. Vegans enjoyed greater protection overall.
- A Taiwanese study of 8,000 vegetarians and vegans showed they had a better metabolic profile – lower blood pressure, better waist circumference and lower BMI – than non-vegetarians.

Of course, studies don't tell the whole story: we're all individuals. An unhealthy veggie diet can be just as poor as a carnivorous one. There *are* steps that vegans in particular need to take to ensure their diet contains essential nutrients, which I list from page 26.

But a well-balanced vegetarian or vegan diet is likely to be:

- Higher in fresh vegetables and fruit;
- Higher in wholegrains, legumes/beans, nuts and seeds;
- Higher in fibre;

- More diverse in both fresh produce and spices, which contain a range of health-promoting antioxidants, vitamins and other nutrients;
- Lower in processed foods (and free from processed meats).

A good veggie/vegan diet shares many features found in the much-researched Mediterranean diet, which is followed by people across southern Europe. Typically it includes lots of vegetables and fruit, pulses/legumes, nuts, grains, some cheese and yogurt, and little red meat: olive oil is usually the main fat used in salads, food preparation and cooking. These communities have been studied extensively by researchers because they have lower rates of heart disease, dementia and cancer than those in other Western countries, and live longer and healthier lives.

The Florence team mentioned above are currently comparing the effectiveness of veggie vs. Mediterranean diets in preventing heart disease in their CARDIVEG study.

Value for money

Eating veggie is cheaper; it's more expensive to rear animals for meat than to grow crops, which is why meat costs more. Also, if you focus on seasonal vegetables and fruit, you'll be eating not only what's **plentiful but it will also be better value** – street markets and stalls in particular adjust their prices when there's a glut, whether it's apples, courgettes or potatoes. Check eatseasonably.co.uk for guidance on what's best to buy now.

Animal welfare concerns

Many vegetarians simply don't want to eat animals. That was my reason for cutting out meat, aged 18. I couldn't see an ethical difference between eating livestock such as pigs or sheep, for example, and eating cats or dogs.

Vegans take it to the next level, and don't consume dairy, eggs or any other foods that derive from animals, such as honey.

If you do still include dairy or eggs in your diet and animal welfare is a concern for you, you will probably want to think carefully about how the animals producing these foods are reared and treated. For example, even though animals may not be killed for milk, male calves born to cows in dairy farms may be culled as they are not needed.

Overall, though, it's much easier now to find ingredients with higher welfare standards than it was when I first became a veggie. Free-range eggs, for example, are seen by most of us as a minimum welfare standard. If we use the money we save by eating less meat to buy some organic or fairly-traded foods, we can also contribute to **better treatment of workers and animals**, rely less on pesticides, and potentially help reduce the use of antibiotics and hormones in animals raised for dairy or eggs.

There's more guidance on this topic on page 320, 5:2 Know-how Fast Day shopping tips.

Environmental and agricultural reasons

Many vegetarians and vegans believe a **vegetable-based diet has less impact on the environment** and **can feed more people**. It takes more effort, money and land to raise animals for meat than it does to grow vegetables.

One study by a team at Oxford University concluded that a global switch to diets that rely less on meat and more on fruit and vegetables could save up to 8 million people from starvation or global warming by 2050, reduce greenhouse gas emissions by two-thirds, and save $1.5 trillion in healthcare/climate-change-related costs, with the most dramatic results coming if we were all to adopt a vegan diet. The claim may sound overblown, but it's food for thought.

Even the most dedicated, optimistic veggie knows the world is unlikely to turn vegetarian or vegan overnight, but shifting towards eating less meat does mean that as individuals our choices are being noted by manufacturers and farmers, bringing about more gradual changes.

Religious reasons

Many faiths advise abstinence of certain meats, either permanently or during certain fasting or observance times. The non-violent credo of Jainism, which seeks to avoid unnecessary injury even to plants, is the most restrictive, while many Hindus and Sikhs avoid all meats, and certain groups of Christians and Muslims also encourage vegetarianism.

It's the taste...

Finally, many of us simply **prefer the flavour of plant-based foods**. I didn't enjoy red meat or strong-flavoured fish before I became a veggie.

Going veggie frees us from the idea that a meal means 'meat and two veg', which can encourage us to try more varied produce, spices and international recipes. Eating out as a veggie can also be exciting, if occasionally challenging – the chefs and cooks who take vegetable cuisine seriously produce some of the most innovative food around.

From the earthy legume dishes of the Middle East to tangy miso from Japan, and the hearty grains that fuel people in northern Europe, there's so much to enjoy: I've used all these influences in developing the Fast Day recipes in this book. Including a range of spices and produce also means we're consuming lots of phytonutrients which help the body work more efficiently and prevent disease. There's never been a better time to enjoy the best of veggie and vegan food.

Vegan, veggie, pescetarian, omnivore… what's the difference?

There are many different approaches to a plant-focused diet; here are some of the main ones.

A vegan avoids all meat, fish and animal products: that includes dairy produce, eggs and honey. In the UK, the Vegan Society says that more than 1 per cent of the population are vegan, and that numbers have grown by 360 per cent in a decade, with 542,000 vegans in 2016 compared to 150,000 in 2006.

The Vegan Society's definition of veganism is: *A philosophy and way of living which seeks to exclude – as far as is possible and practicable – all forms of exploitation of, and cruelty to, animals for food, clothing or any other purpose.* This includes not using certain cosmetics and household products that may have been tested on animals, and avoiding visiting zoos or circuses with animals.

A vegetarian avoids all meat, poultry and fish. Sometimes I explain it by saying I don't eat 'anything with a face'. A lacto-ovo vegetarian eats milk-based foods and eggs. In the UK, studies suggest up to 12 per cent of the population are either veggie or follow a mainly vegetarian diet. Worldwide, it's estimated that up to 375 million people follow a vegetarian diet for religious, ethical or health reasons: the highest percentage is found in India, followed by Israel, the UK and the Netherlands.

Many vegetarians also avoid wearing leather, or using products tested on animals. In this book, we use the word **'veggie'** to mean vegetarian.

'Pescatarians' are vegetarians who eat fish but not meat/poultry. Many restaurants still offer a fish dish as a vegetarian option, which can be annoying for those of us who don't eat fish.

Omnivores don't avoid any foods, but many people *are* now trying to eat more plant-based meals and minimise their consumption of meat for one or more of the reasons above. The rise of Meat-free Mondays, for example, reveals the increasing interest in eating less meat. A Mintel survey in 2013 found that 12 per cent of people in the UK were vegetarian, while 23 per cent were reducing the amount of meat in their diet. If you're trying this out, you might call yourself a **demi-vegetarian,** or a **flexigan**! You can also reduce your meat intake gradually, with a view to becoming vegetarian or even vegan in the long term. Fast Days would be an obvious place to begin.

Nutrition for veggies and vegans

Eating well as a vegetarian and vegan is not a problem, but vegans in particular need to take extra care that their diets include some essential vitamins that don't naturally occur in plant-based foods.

Our food intake should supply both '**macro-nutrients**' – fuel, in the form of fat, protein and carbohydrate – and '**micro-nutrients**' – which are vitamins, minerals and compounds that are needed for the body to function properly. Here's a simple guide to making sure your body gets what it needs.

Macro nutrients

Fat

'**Is fat good or bad for me?**' is one of the biggest questions in nutrition at present. For years, governments have advised us to eat a diet that's lower in all fats, but especially saturated fat (butter, dairy, coconut oil). Yet obesity levels have soared worldwide since that advice was adopted, and some of the studies recommending a low-fat diet for health have been challenged.

The fats we eat are higher in calories than either carbohydrates or protein: fat contains 9 calories per gram, while carbohydrates and protein contain only 4. We store excess energy as fat, but that energy can come from eating fat, carbs or proteins. Fat inside our bodies also cushions our organs, keeps us warm and allows us to absorb vitamins that are only 'fat-soluble' (vitamins A, D, E and K). Some fats – omega 3 and 6 essential fatty acids – need to be taken in via food because we can't make them ourselves. These help the brain, the immune system and your heart and circulation, and consuming the right ratio takes planning, especially if you don't eat fish (see omega 3 and 6, page 37).

Fat also helps to make food taste good, and adds that succulent 'mouth feel' that makes food seem to melt in the mouth.

Fats are classified according to their chemical structure – that's where the labels of saturated, monounsaturated and polyunsaturated come from. Saturated fats are mostly solid at room temperature (such as butter and coconut oil), while the others (unsaturated fats) are liquid at room temperature, such as oils.

The subject of fat is controversial, and research is emerging all the time, making it difficult to offer hard and fast rules on what and how much you should eat. Saturated and unsaturated fats have the same number of calories per gram (energy density) so will have the same effect on trying to lose weight. At the moment, the UK government recommends that we limit our saturated fat intake to less than 20g per day for women and 30g a day for men. Trans fats should be limited to less than 5g per day for adults.

What I can do is tell you what I do: I include saturated fat – butter and coconut oil – in my diet, especially for cooking, but I do keep an eye on how much I use because of its energy density. I definitely avoid hydrogenated fats or trans fats, which are turned into solids via an industrial process and are bad for human health. Avoid these in both cooking and processed foods: check for the words 'hydrogenated' or 'partially hydrogenated' on the label.

Culinary oils are almost all vegan: olive oil, groundnut oil, rapeseed and sesame oil all have benefits particularly for your heart. I don't use oils labelled 'vegetable oils', which are usually corn or soya, because the production methods are highly industrial, their fatty acid ratios are not helpful, and they don't have the nutritional benefits of olive or nut oils.

Coconut oil is solid at room temperature, and, unusually for a non-animal product, is a saturated fat. It contains anti-microbial lauric acid, which is rich in medium-chain triglycerides, a form of fat that our bodies and brains find easier to use as fuel. I like it best in fried or grilled Asian and Indian dishes to complement the mild coconut flavour. Bear in mind the government guidance about saturated fats above.

Other **saturated fats are usually animal-derived:** butter and ghee are made from milk, so are acceptable for lacto-ovo vegetarians, but lard, goose fat and suet are by-products of meat production, so are not suitable.

Other sources of dietary fat for veggies include dairy products such as cheese and yogurt, and for both veggies and vegans, avocados, nuts and seeds.

What to cook with: I use extra-virgin olive oil for dressing salads and when frying or grilling at low temperatures (it's not stable at higher temperatures). I use butter, rapeseed oil, groundnut oil or coconut oil for baking and frying at higher temperatures.

Protein

Protein is often called the '**building block**' macronutrient because the amino acids it contains help the body grow and repair itself.

There are 21 kinds of amino acids; the body can manufacture 12 of them (though some only very slowly) while nine need to be obtained from food sources – these are known as the 'essential amino acids'. A food is a complete protein when it contains an adequate proportion of these nine amino acids.

For **vegetarians, dairy and eggs offer complete proteins in a single 'package'**, as do quinoa and soya; while products made from **fermented soya, such as tofu and tempeh, are good vegan options.** Quorn is also useful for vegetarians, but not for vegans, because it is produced using egg.

If you're vegan, you'll find many **combinations of food will produce 'complete' proteins;** for example, rice with beans or peas, or hummus (containing chickpeas and sesame seeds). Research used to suggest vegans *had* to eat these at the same meal, but now we know it is just as effective if they are all eaten within the space of a day or two.

Protein can make you feel fuller, so you eat less. Eating enough protein also helps to reduce the amount of lean tissue (muscle) that is lost through dieting.

So how much protein should you eat? If our bodies use proteins to grow and repair, then surely eating plenty of it is a good thing?

It's a question of balance: too much *animal* protein may be damaging because it over-stimulates these bodily processes. In one interesting but controversial study, middle-aged people (50–64 years old) eating diets high in animal (meat and dairy) proteins had a higher risk of premature death and four times the risk of dying of cancer as those who ate a lower-protein diet. But plant proteins, such as those in lentils and beans, did not show the same risks. Also, over the age of 65, **higher-protein diets seemed to be protective against early death**, perhaps because ageing bodies need more help in repairing damage.

The NHS in the UK recommends men consume around 55.5g of protein per day and women around 45g: as an example, a medium egg has around 6g of protein, a 50g serving of full-fat Greek yogurt has 5g, a 100g serving of tofu around 8g, and a 50g serving of quinoa, around 6.5g. On a Fast Day, when levels of other macro-nutrients are lower, you may not achieve that level, but do aim to include some protein in every meal.

Carbohydrate

Carbohydrates are sugars, starches and fibre found in plants and dairy products: plants actually produce starches and sugar to store energy, through photosynthesis.

Carbs get a bad press, yet many of the healthiest foods in our diet – high-fibre green leafy vegetables, for example – are carbohydrates. In fact, it is not the carbs themselves but how some carbs are processed and prepared by us that can make them unhealthy.

Our bodies **use carbohydrates for energy**, producing glucose for immediate use, and glycogen, which is stored in the liver and muscles to be used when the body needs extra energy rapidly – a bit like a reserve tank of petrol.

The big difference is between simple carbohydrates (sugars), which are digested very quickly, and complex carbs (vegetables and grains), which take longer for the body to break down. Industrial processing – for example, turning beets into sugar –

converts complex carbs into simple ones, and strips out many of the micronutrients we need.

Blood sugar questions

Insulin plays a key role in how our bodies function; the hormone controls how our bodies use sugars/carbohydrates, and regulates blood sugar levels. One of the biggest health threats from obesity globally is type 2 diabetes, when the body either stops secreting enough insulin or stops reacting to it as strongly – or both. Glucose then builds up in the body, causing serious damage that can include heart disease, blindness and nerve damage and can even lead to amputations, especially of the lower limbs.

From a weight-loss point of view, we also need to know that **when insulin levels are high, we can't burn fat**. It's one of the reasons why leaving gaps between eating, and avoiding snacking, may be more effective than reducing calories alone.

Sugary foods and processed carbohydrates generally can cause a 'spike' in insulin, followed by a crash where we feel unwell. So, do we need to avoid all food with sugars in it? Or even all carbohydrates?

The key is to eat balanced meals, which contain protein, fat and complex carbohydrates, as these macronutrients are digested at different rates, so we avoid a crash. The exceptions – very sugary foods, sweets and, most of all, fizzy drinks – should be severely limited.

But **avoiding all carbs is not a good idea:** many whole grains and vegetables are high in micronutrients and fibre. Whole grains – including the wheat products that many health-food gurus urge us to cut out – also contain 'resistant starches', which help us feel fuller, and have positive effects on digestion, eye and brain health, and our response to insulin.

Eating food that is as whole and unprocessed as possible is important: compare eating one whole orange, with lots of fibre, to drinking a glass of orange juice. The former takes a while to eat, and contains fibre that slows its digestion. The latter can be drunk in a few seconds and increases blood sugar levels without the fibre to slow it down.

As a rule, I avoid 'drinking my calories', except for that Mediterranean favourite, red wine…

Reducing sugar consumption is a good idea for the reasons given above. 'Natural sugars' such as honey and agave may have been produced on a smaller scale than refined sugars, but they still have a very similar effect on the body. Agave and honey are sweeter than sugar, which means you can use a little less than table sugar. These natural sweeteners, plus molasses and maple syrup, do contain traces of micronutrients such as potassium and calcium, but at such low levels that you'd have to consume enormous quantities to feel the benefit. Do use sparingly if you like the taste, but table sugar is cheaper, of course.

Sweeteners are useful *and* controversial. There are numerous scare stories online about their potential dangers, though most have been extensively tested for toxicity. A greater concern is their wider effects on the body.

I used to have low-sugar fizzy drinks with sweeteners once or twice a week, but I now only drink them occasionally. There are question marks around whether a sweetener may make us crave sweeter foods, or affect our insulin response. A recent study found an association between drinking more than two fizzy drinks sweetened either with sugar or artificial sweeteners every day, and the risk of developing type 2 diabetes. The Swedish researchers suggested the sweetened drinks could be affecting insulin resistance. As usual, it's not clear-cut, as the consumption might be part of a generally unhealthy lifestyle, or simply a sign of the increased thirst that often accompanies the onset of the disease.

In addition, I am unsure of their effect on our gut bacteria – a new area of research that is giving us a brand-new insight into how we digest food and how that affects our health. Overall, I'd say sweeteners don't add anything beneficial, but they *may* help you wean yourself off drinking lots of sugary drinks – but avoid too many, and keep an eye on the research!

The gluten question

Gluten is a separate issue, though it's often talked about in the context of starchy carbs like bread and other common grains. That's because wheat, barley and rye contain the mix of proteins known as gluten. Found in wheat and some other wholegrains, it gives elasticity to dough and makes bread chewy. But gluten is a serious health risk for coeliacs, because their immune system attacks it, causing 'collateral' damage to the intestine. The condition is diagnosed through a blood test.

Even if we're not coeliac, some of us do find that **too much gluten in our diet appears to cause us bloating or digestive problems**. If that's the case, you may prefer to try 'ancient grains' like emmer wheat or spelt, or build your diet around other grains such as rice or oats, or 'pseudo-grains' such as quinoa and buckwheat. But if you want to exclude any food group, I'd suggest you seek advice from a registered dietician first.

Micronutrients and phytonutrients

Micronutrients are also found in what we eat – we need them, but in smaller amounts. These include **vitamins such as A, C and D, minerals such as iron or calcium, and anti-oxidants/phytonutrients found in plants** that may reduce the risk of ageing or disease.

There are a number of micronutrients that vegans and vegetarians need to take care to include in their diet.

B12

This vitamin is essential for brain function, the production of red blood cells, healthy nerve function and more: deficiency can be dangerous and cause pernicious anaemia, nerve damage and low mood. It is found naturally in animal products, including dairy and eggs. Vegans obtain it through fortified foods – such as cereals or nutritional yeast (see page 325) – but you may also like to consider taking a supplement or using a spray.

Calcium

Calcium is a mineral that strengthens teeth and bones, and it also plays a part in the nervous system, muscles and blood clotting. Dairy products are a good source, and for vegans, it's found in green leafy vegetables and grains. Wheat flour and some dairy milk alternatives will be fortified with calcium too.

Iron

Iron is another mineral needed for haemoglobin, which transports oxygen around the body. Leafy vegetables, egg yolk, dried fruits, nuts, cereal grains and fortified cereals (ideally with no added sugar) are good sources. Ingesting iron along with vitamin C helps absorption, so combine iron-rich foods with colourful fruit or veg. For example, serve unsweetened bran or oat-based breakfast cereal with fresh fruit, bean-based soup with veggies, or peanut butter on toast with sliced apple.

Zinc

Zinc helps us heal after injury and aids production of the enzymes that support good digestion. Dairy produce, eggs, legumes or beans, tofu, grains, nuts and seeds are all good sources. However, vegans do need to ensure they're eating enough foods rich in zinc because a diet higher in unrefined grains may block the absorption of some of the mineral.

Antioxidants and phytonutrients

You may have heard of antioxidants, which are used to promote everything from fruit juice to face cream. Antioxidants reduce 'oxidative stress' or, to put it simply, the damage caused to cells by oxygen and the accompanying 'free radicals'.

Antioxidants were hailed as the ultimate anti-ageing cure, but clinical trials haven't borne that out. Very high doses of vitamins or minerals with antioxidant properties – such as vitamin C or E – either had no effect on disease prevention or even increased the risk. It may be that taking supplements, rather than consuming micronutrients through food, misses out vital other elements: again, a varied, wholefood diet is likely to be better.

Phytonutrients are found in plants – they're what give them their many colours but, more importantly, they also affect how our bodies work. There may be up to 20,000 of them, and they have very different effects, many of which are only now being studied or discovered (though traditional diets and medicines often make use of them, suggesting their benefits may have been recognised long ago).

Here are some you may have heard of:

Nutrient	Found in	Possible benefits for
Anthocyanins	red and purple berries, onions, potatoes	blood vessels/circulation
Beta-carotene	orange and green produce including pumpkins, sweet potatoes, apricots, kale and broccoli	immune system, vision, skin and bone health
Lutein	egg yolks, mustard, corn, courgettes	eye health
Lycopene	tomatoes, red peppers, watermelons	heart, reducing prostate cancer risk

Resveratrol	red wine, grapes, peanuts	heart and lungs, reducing damaging inflammation, protecting against cancer
Sulforaphane	broccoli, other cruciferous vegetables	inhibiting cancer growth and development

You'll notice that different-coloured produce tends to have different properties – the common advice to 'eat a rainbow of different-coloured foods' is not just about the foods looking good on the plate! The great thing about a veggie and vegan diet is that we tend to eat a range of different plant foods to keep it varied, so we're getting a good selection of these chemicals. Spices are also very good sources of concentrated phytonutrients; for example, curcumin, found in turmeric, is being extensively studied for its potential to both prevent and inhibit the growth of cancer cells.

One other thing to note is that resveratrol may mimic the effect of fasting by reducing inflammation and improving cell function. And in both cases, part of the effect may come from the activation of **sirtuins**, which regulate metabolism and other functions. The SIRT diet that gained attention in 2015 includes foods that aim to activate sirtuins, including turmeric (again!), olive oil, green veg and soya – all of which can be enjoyed in a vegan or veggie diet.

Omega 3 and 6 fatty acids
Omega 6 (linoleic acid) and omega 3 (alpha-linoleic acid) can't be produced by the body but are essential fatty acids,

needed for good health. Having the balance of the two is also important, and getting it right can be difficult for omnivores and veggies alike. Veggies and vegans generally will consume plenty of omega 6 (found in vegetables, fruits, soya and grains), but it's very important to make the effort to include sources of omega 3 too. Most omnivores will consume omega 3 through fish oils, so if you're veggie, try other sources such as ground flaxseeds or chia seeds, which you can sprinkle on yogurt or savoury dishes: cook or make dressings with rapeseed oil, or include walnuts in salads. Seaweed is the only vegan source of long-chain omega 3 fatty acids, which are particularly good for your heart (try the Sesame sea vegetable salad, page 270, or buy ground seaweed to sprinkle over other savoury foods).

Supplements

It's always better to get the micronutrients you need from food, but I think a good supplement can be a useful insurance policy for vegetarians and especially vegans. You can buy supplements specifically designed to address nutrients that may be lacking in your diet, or review your own diet and pick those that seem most useful to you. Look for supplements that do not contain gelatine, which is sometimes used as a coating for capsules.

I confess to a personal interest here, I recently – and unexpectedly – found through a blood test that my B12 levels were on the low side, even though I eat plenty of dairy. The research shows that B12 deficiency is not only about what you eat, but how able your body is to absorb it. I now take a sublingual supplement – it melts under the tongue, so the vitamin is absorbed more efficiently than it can be through food. I definitely feel more energetic, though I know that may partly be the placebo effect.

Recent guidance from the UK government suggests that everyone in the country should take a vitamin D supplement of 10µg per day. Vitamin D is made in our skin when exposed to sunshine, but covering up against the sun's harmful rays, working indoors and not getting enough fresh air is making us deficient.

Special groups and needs

Pregnant and breastfeeding women

This book is about combining veggie and vegan food with intermittent fasting, and fasting is NOT advised during pregnancy or while breastfeeding. A vegetarian or vegan diet is suitable for pregnant and nursing women, but you're strongly advised to take advice from your doctor or midwife to ensure you are getting all the nutrients that you and your growing baby need. The Vegan Society has a great section on nutrition: www.vegansociety.com.

Children and teenagers

Again, this book isn't aimed at children or teenagers who are growing: fasting is not advised for those groups. Bringing up veggie children has become a lot easier in recent years, but as children do need high-energy food and a full range of nutrients as they grow, you need to be well informed to make the best choices. The Vegan Society website contains lots of useful resources, or you can speak to your GP, Health Visitor or a registered dietician.

Older adults

As we age, our ability to absorb and use nutrients may decrease. Our energy needs tend to reduce, too, and sometimes our appetite, often because we slowly lose some of our ability to smell and taste. However our requirement for protein increases.

Maintaining your intake of protein and all the micronutrients in this section is very important, along with staying active and spending time outdoors to keep vitamin D levels topped up.

Unexpected item in the veggie area: hidden animal ingredients

You know what you should include in your diet, but what should you avoid? Here are a few non-veggie ingredients to avoid when you are shopping or eating out.

Gelatine

Gelatine is a gelling agent that is used in mousses, desserts, some sweets and some savoury dishes to give a firm 'set'; it's made from collagen, extracted from animals, so is not suitable for vegetarians. If a dish wobbles, and is not specifically labelled as veggie, chances are it includes gelatine; it is also used in some yogurts.

Veggie alternatives include agar-agar and carrageenan, both derived from types of seaweed.

Rennet

Rennet is used in some hard cheeses to help the proteins in milk form a curd. It can either be made from animal sources or can be wholly vegetarian. Most supermarket cheeses now specify on the labels whether they're vegetarian or not, but some specific, often traditional, cheeses must be made with animal rennet, such as Parmesan, so I'd suggest using Grana Padano, which usually is vegetarian and tastes very similar. It's also often cheaper.

Animal stocks

A vegetable soup often seems the ideal way to start a meal if you're veggie, but double-check that the stock is vegetable-based. Many restaurants will use chicken or beef stock for a richer flavour, especially in French onion soup, where it's seen as an essential ingredient.

Lard or solid animal fats in baked goods/fried foods

Lard, suet, dripping, beef or goose fat may be used in traditional sauces, baked goods (such as lardy cake or some brands of tortilla) or even to fry chips in upmarket burger bars.

Veggie food cooked alongside meat

Most vegetarians would prefer not to have their food cooked in the same pan or on the same grill as meat. If this is something that you care about, do ask about cooking practices in restaurants – apart from anything else, it will raise awareness for the chefs about what's important to veggie customers.

Invisible animal foods

These include red cochineal food colouring (made from beetles, but less frequently used now), Worcestershire sauce (contains anchovies: look for the veggie versions), fish sauce in Thai and Asian cooking (hard to avoid in some curries or curry pastes: check the label) and isinglass in real ale and some wines (a fish product used to clarify liquids). Again, the best thing to do is ask waiting staff about what is in the food if you're eating out, or read the nutritional info on packets when you are shopping.

Supplements can also contain animal products, for example, fish oils rather than flaxseed. Again, look for those marked as vegetarian or vegan-friendly.

This list may sound intimidating, but the good news is that as vegetarianism and veganism continues to be more widely adopted, manufacturers and chefs are becoming more aware of our needs, and are looking for animal-free alternatives.

How to fast

Over the next few pages you'll find a brief guide to fasting. If you already do 5:2, you can dive right into the recipes, starting on page 57.

Getting started with 5:2

It's simple to get started with 5:2. Here's what you need to do:

1 Set your weight-loss (or maintenance) goal and Fast Day limits.
2 Pick two days on which you will fast in the week ahead – they don't have to be the same days each week, and they don't have to be two consecutive days (see page 49).
3 Plan your meals to fit your calorie limit on those fasting days.

Important: it's always advisable to talk to your doctor before making big changes to your diet. Many GPs are now very supportive of intermittent fasting and 5:2. If you have a chronic health condition, or take medication, you should definitely talk to them before starting (see page 5).

1: Set your weight-loss goal and Fast Day limits

Record your current measurements

- Weigh yourself and use this measurement along with your height to check your BMI (Body Mass Index) using the chart on page 365 or the calculator at www.the5-2dietbook.com/calculator. Weighing yourself twice a week has been shown to help people trying to lose weight, probably by keeping your motivation up! Weighing yourself too regularly is not helpful, as it is likely to show small fluctuations due to water weight.

- Measure your hips, waist, chest/bust and, if you like, your upper arms and thighs at their widest point. Calculate your waist–height ratio by dividing your waist measurement by your height in either centimetres or inches.

- If you prefer not to weigh yourself regularly, you could find clothes that are tight and try them on instead – you can then check progress quickly by trying these on again.

- You could also take a photograph of how you look now: you never have to show it to anyone else but it can be very motivating as you lose weight.

Evaluating your results

BMI: if your BMI is over 25kg/m^2 (or 23kg/m^2 for some ethnic groups) you're classed as overweight: the higher the figure, the higher your potential risk of health problems due to your weight. It's a very general indicator: it doesn't work well for sports people or bodybuilders, for example, as they have a greater muscle mass than average.

Waist/hip ratio: the bigger your waist, the more likely you are to have 'visceral' fat around vital organs, which is a risk factor for heart disease and type 2 diabetes. You're at greater risk if your waist (measured midway between the bottom of your ribcage and your hipbone) is **more than half of your height: that means a figure of over 0.5.**

For example, here are my own measurements, starting with the ones I took just before I first began 5:2 and ending with those I took when I reached my optimal weight:

August 2012: Waist (32 inches/81cm) ÷ Height (64 inches/162cm) = 0.5 (so borderline)

January 2013: Waist (29.5in/75cm) ÷ Height (64in/162cm) = 0.46

April 2013: Waist (27.5in/70cm) ÷ Height (64in/162cm) = 0.43

If you're shocked to see your own measurements written down, I understand – I've been there. But remember, you're taking the first step to making things better.

Set your goal

Whether you want to lose weight or maintain the weight you're at, you need a goal. Here are some possible objectives.

- A weight that puts you just into 'healthy' BMI category (so, between $23kg/m^2$ and $25kg/m^2$, depending on your ethnic background).

- The weight at which you feel most happy and confident.
- The size you were on your wedding day, for example, or another significant time when you felt that you were in great shape.

You might also set mini-goals to keep you motivated. For example:

- Moving from the obese to overweight category in the BMI chart.
- Reaching the 15- (210-lb), 12- (168-lb) or 10-stone (140-lb) mark.
- Fitting into a favourite pair of jeans.
- Losing 5–10% of your total body weight. This is associated with big increases in health, even if it doesn't get you within the BMI category, so could be a great place to start.

Set your Fast Day calorie limit

5:2 is based on creating a **deficit or 'calorie gap' between the energy your body uses and the energy you consume.** If you create a gap, your body will burn excess fat as fuel, and you'll lose weight.

Always remember that losing weight too quickly will mean you are more likely to put weight back on; this is called the 'adiposity rebound'. It is best to make any weight loss slow and maintainable. For sustainable weight loss, we're aiming at 1–2lbs (0.45–1kg) per week. Studies suggest you need a deficit of around 3,500 calories to lose one pound (0.45kg) in weight so the Fast Day limits should produce that deficit for most of us.

The guideline for Fast Days is **around 500 calories (or under) per day if you're a woman, or 600 (or under) if you're a man.** This is based on the energy needs for an average adult: so, if you eat a normal, healthy balanced diet on the other days, the Fast Days will produce a calorie gap of 3,000–3,600 calories per week.

In 2017, Dr Michael Mosley, who presented the inspirational BBC *Horizon* programme about intermittent fasting in 2012, wrote that an **800 calorie limit** rather than 500–600 isn't going to make that much of a difference, particularly if you go low carb on the other 5 days.

There are pros and cons to this: it may be **less daunting if you find 500–600 leaves you too hungry on Fast Days.** The cons might include the calorie reduction slightly **reducing the pace of weight loss** (especially if you have a slower metabolism/lower energy needs), and perhaps the less strict limit making us **less careful/aware** of what we eat on both Fast and non-fasting days.

Why you might want to set a personalised limit
All sorts of factors influence your *actual* energy needs, including:

- Age
- Gender
- How heavy and tall you are
- How active you are in your everyday life
- The composition of your gut bacteria, which affects how efficiently we extract energy from food.

Generally, the larger you are – and the more weight you are carrying – the more calories you need to sustain your current size. If you're a lot heavier than the average, you may therefore find it harder at first to cope with consuming only 500–600 calories per day. You can better understand your overall calorie needs by working out your *Total Daily Energy Expenditure* (TDEE), which takes the factors above into consideration, then you can adjust your Fast Day calorie limit to suit before you get started.

The easiest way to work it out is at www.the5-2dietbook. com/calculator – you might get slightly varied results from different online calculators, but the difference won't be substantial. Once you have your TDEE, divide it by 4 to get your daily limit. So, for example, if your TDEE is 2,900, 725 calories would be the most we'd suggest you eat on a Fast Day. It's just an estimate, but it's a useful one.

(TDEE can also be a useful tool for non-fasting days, to help you check you're not eating much more or less than your body needs to function well. For more guidance, see **Part 3: Eating Well for Life**.)

NB: The TDEE is calculated by combining your activity levels with your *Basal Metabolic Rate* (BMR), which estimates what your body needs for only the most basic bodily functions. **Always use the TDEE and not BMR** to guide your calorie consumption.

2: Pick two Fast Days for the week ahead

Look at your diary and choose two days to fast in the week ahead. A Fast Day lasts from the last meal the previous day until breakfast the day after. For example:

Sunday: Eat dinner/last meal of the day at normal time, e.g. 7pm

Monday: Fast – eat up to 500–600 calories, over no more than three meals

Tuesday: Eat breakfast/first meal of the day at your normal time, e.g. 8am

Which days should I choose?

- Separate your Fast Days at first. For example, fast on Monday and Wednesday, or Tuesday and Thursday. It's easier to stick to your limit when you know that tomorrow you can eat what you like.
- Once you're used to fasting, you can do a 'back to back'; i.e. two days in succession.
- For your first fasts, choose days when you're busy but not under serious work or family pressure.
- You can change days each week to suit your diary.
- You can do more than two fasts in a week (4:3). This will increase the calorie gap and may speed up weight loss, but avoid doing more than two fasts back to back and make sure you are not trying to lose weight too quickly or you will reduce your fat-free mass, which will have a negative inpact on your BMR.

3: Plan your Fast Day

The final stage is to plan what you're going to eat, and when. The more organised you are, the less likely you are to go over your limit, or abandon your Fast Day.

When should I eat on Fast Days? And how often?

- You can eat 1–3 small meals on a Fast Day. As I outlined on page 14, leaving longer gaps between eating, or only eating 1 or 2 meals may increase the health benefits of fasting. Many 5:2 dieters began by eating very three small meals, but now skip breakfast or lunch and either eat once or twice instead. Some of us – me included – definitely find that the later we leave it to eat, the less hungry we feel.

- You may want to plan a flexible menu for yourself, bearing in mind you are transitioning from three larger meals every day. For example, perhaps choose two larger dishes to fuel you, with a third dish – a side or salad – that could be eaten any time if you get really hungry on your first couple of fasts (see the Fast Day Meal Plans, starting on page 291, for lots of ideas).

- Some people find water fasts/juice fasts easier. Personally, I prefer to eat solid food, and you should remember that fruit-based juices are high in sugar and sometimes calories, and are also low in fibre and protein. Also, eating fruits or vegetables whole means they're digested more slowly, which staves off hunger pangs for longer. But juice fasts should be safe for one day at a time if you're in good health and not taking medication. Check with your doctor if you have any concerns, though.

Fasting tips and tricks

Your first Fast Day can be exciting, but also unsettling. As we've seen, fasting can help our health by placing us under good stress: like exercising, this way of eating can feel like a stretch at first, until we get used to it and the positive effects it brings.

Our daily lives are often built around meal times, so changing that routine feels odd initially. Plus, many of us have forgotten how it feels to be hungry!

Once you're used to Fast Days, you'll almost certainly feel energetic and positive, and many people get through their first fasts with no unwelcome changes. However, there are a few sensations that you might experience, so here they are, along with suggestions as to how to manage them.

- **Feeling cold** This is common in winter, partly because your body generates more heat when it's digesting food. Try drinking hot drinks and wearing extra layers.
- **Headaches** These are common when making any dietary change due to dehydration and/or changes to blood sugar. This should settle over time, but drinking plenty of water, or taking a mild painkiller, will help. Food contains lots of water, so if you are fasting you will need to drink more to compensate.
- **Irritability** You may feel grumpy at first: that's the lack of blood sugar again. Try to build in a non-food

treat to look forward to: a long hot bath, a hand massage or perhaps your favourite TV show.

- **Digestive changes** As you're not eating as much you may not need to open your bowels as often, or you may find that the next day your digestion is slower (or faster) than normal. Most people find that their digestion settles as they adapt to the new way of eating.

- **Feeling light-headed** This is much less common, but have a small calorie-counted snack on standby on those first days, such as a small handful of nuts or a mini high-protein cereal bar (check nutritional information on the packet – some snacks marketed as healthy can still be high in calories). If you feel very unwell, eat normally and take medical advice before trying a second fast.

Here are some tips to help you adapt, and you can find plenty more on my YouTube video channel: http://bit.ly/1t8aBtr

- **Drink plenty of water, black coffee, tea or low-cal herbal teas.** Milk can affect insulin levels but can still be included in the fast. Diet drinks also may affect insulin and gut bacteria in unhelpful ways so are best avoided (though I occasionally have a diet cola on a Fast Day...).

- **Distract yourself.** Hunger tends to come in waves, so do things that take your mind off it until it subsides. Make yourself a drink, visit the 5:2 Facebook group, phone a friend or read a book.

- **Move more.** Many of us go for a run or to the gym on a Fast Day with no difference in stamina or performance. Just be careful and listen to your body the first couple of times, taking a break if need be, and make sure you stay hydrated. And no, you can't 'earn' extra calories on a Fast Day, but you will feel virtuous afterwards.
- **Feel your hunger.** Remember that it's positive to **relearn what appetite feels like**, and how small meals can still satisfy us.
- **Celebrate food.** When you *do* eat, make an occasion of it if possible. Lay the table, use pretty plates, pour yourself some water and add a slice of lemon, play relaxing music. And savour every bite… eating this way is more satisfying to the senses! It might even teach you to eat more mindfully, which could benefit your dietary habits in the long run.
- **Create a support network.** You're more likely to succeed in making changes to your lifestyle if you have a support network. Try 5:2 with a friend, or explain what you're doing to someone who cares about you. Our Facebook group is also super supportive, and it's a closed group so posts won't be visible to friends on your timeline: www.facebook. com/groups/the52diet.
- Finally, remember the 5:2 catchphrase: '**Tomorrow you can eat what you like**'. Though most of us find the next day we're not that hungry!

Frequently asked quesions

How quickly will I lose weight?

In our large Facebook group, most people who are fasting to slim down will lose **1–2lb (0.45–1kg) per week**. Some lose a lot more, especially in the first few weeks. Weight varies a lot day by day – hormonal changes in women can add 5–6lb (2.2–2.75kg), or in a few cases even 10lb (4.5kg) or more at different times of the month! I recommend weighing yourself at the same time and on the same day each week. I found it motivating to weigh myself the morning after the second fast of the week.

In general, people with more weight to lose are likely to see more rapid losses, and the last few pounds to your target can be the toughest to shift.

What if I'm not losing weight?

If after a couple of weeks of following this plan you're not losing weight, it may be that the amount you're **eating on your non-fasting days is cancelling out the calorie gap** produced by the fasts. There's lots more advice on non-fasting days in Part 3, but if you're not losing, start by **carefully adding up the calories you're consuming on two typical average non-fasting days**, perhaps a weekday and a weekend day.

You want to be roughly around your TDEE (see page 46). If you're not, consider **reducing your portion size and cutting down on snacks or drinks between meals** to bring it into line. Your TDEE is plenty to keep you full and satisfied.

You could also consider **switching to 4:3** for a couple of weeks, to see if that kick-starts weight loss.

If **you've lost a lot of weight, your TDEE will reduce,** so recalculate it after every 7lb/3kg to make sure you're aware of how many calories you need on non-fasting days. Alternatively, you can offset any reduction by becoming more active, to push your energy needs up again.

Certain **medical conditions**, including hypothyroidism, can make it harder to shift weight, so if you are confident you are following the plan correctly, it's worth discussing your situation with your GP.

Checklist – are you ready to 5:2?

- Do you have a goal – either weight loss or maintenance?
- Have you chosen your first Fast Day?
- Do you know how often and when you will eat on that day?

Great stuff! Now, let's see what's on the menu…

2

THE

5:2

RECIPES

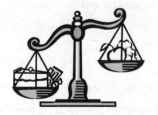

What do you want to eat today? In this section you'll find over 80 fantastic vegetarian and vegan recipes. As a 5:2 veggie myself, the dishes I've included here are the ones that I love – filling, colourful and packed with flavour. They make fasting as enjoyable as it is good for you. For this book, I've discovered some new favourite ingredients, recreated classics to make them fast-friendly and tested them all out on friends, family and neighbours.

You'll also find inspiring 5:2 stories alongside some of these recipes, from people who've had incredible results by combining fasting with veggie and vegan food.

Notes on recipes

Calories: All recipes are calorie-counted, but please note that many processed or branded ingredients goods vary in calorie content. The totals in this book use the lowest-calorie option. For example, different brands of strained Greek yogurts range from between 95 and 130 calories per 100ml, so we'll be using 95 calories to determine the calorie count in a recipe. For more on calorie counts and how they've been calculated, see the guide on page 344.

Butter vs oil: Where butter or oil are both suitable in a recipe, as a vegetarian I use butter as it's fractionally lower in calories and I love the flavour. If you're vegan, most oils have similar calorie counts – see the guidance on page 346. To cut calories further, you can also use a branded low-calorie cooking spray, but please check the label first to see the energy content. Or you can fill a small spray bottle with half oil and half water to spray over your cooking pan, shaking well before each use and wiping the nozzle clear when needed.

Suitability: The following are used to indicate which recipes are suitable for different diets:

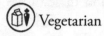 Vegetarian

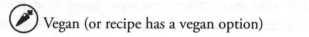 Vegan (or recipe has a vegan option)

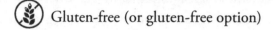 Gluten-free (or gluten-free option)

CHAPTER ONE

Brunch

Brunch is one of my favourite meals – and these dishes are well worth getting out of bed for. Whether you want to take a bowlful of warming cinnamon porridge to work with you, or treat your family to tacos for a leisurely weekend meal with the Sunday papers, these satisfying meals work any time, any place, anywhere. Don't forget that lots of 5:2ers – me included – have found skipping breakfast actually makes us *less* hungry. So simply enjoy these dishes whatever time you fancy!

RECIPES

HERBY WILD MUSHROOM PARCEL, ⓘ⊘⊛, 155

INDIAN CHILLI BREAKFAST PANCAKES, ⓘ⊘⊛, 120 per pancake

HOMEMADE BAKED BEANS ON TOAST, ⓘ⊘⊛, 195

AUSSIE SMOOTHIE WITH AVOCADO, KIWI
AND PINK GRAPEFRUIT, ⓘ⊘⊛, 169

BAKED AVOCADO STUFFED WITH BEANS
AND SMOKED CHEESE, ⓘ⊛, 209

SPICED BRUNCH SCRAMBLE, ⓘ⊘⊛, 159

PEA AND HERB PANCAKES WITH WATERCRESS
AND POACHED EGGS, ⓘ⊛, 222

FRESH CORN AND BLACK BEAN TACOS, ⓘ⊘⊛, 247

YOGURT-BAKED TRUFFLED EGGS WITH GREEN LEAVES, ⓘ⊛, 247

CINNAMON BUCKWHEAT PORRIDGE WITH FIG
AND STRAWBERRIES, ⓘ⊘⊛, 245

5:2 Lives

KAREN'S HEALTH MAKEOVER

'Fasting is as natural as breathing now.'

Before: feeling frumpy
After: size 8 jeans

Karen Hill first noticed it was harder to stay in shape when she hit her forties. Initially, going to the gym was enough, but that didn't last. 'The weight started to creep on again, probably through making bad food choices and starting the menopause. I hate feeling uncomfortable and the extra weight did not sit well with me.'

Karen, who is now 54, saw the *Horizon* documentary about intermittent fasting, but couldn't find much information about the practicalities of the diet. 'A few months later I was browsing Amazon and I saw Kate's first book about 5:2 and bought it. While reading the book, I thought, she's just had a ready-made side dish for her fast, that's easy, I can do this. I think I really wanted the health benefits, too, which would be a bonus if I lost my excess weight.'

Karen decided to start her first fast in early January 2013. 'I was excited before my first fasts. I planned them for a Monday and Thursday as they are my busiest days at work. I remember that food was constantly on my mind during my first Fast Days. But the feelings the day after a Fast Day were remarkable – how empowered I felt.'

From that first day to now, Karen has come down three dress sizes and lost at least two stone (28lb), though as she doesn't own scales, she goes by the fit of her clothes. 'I was in a very tight 12 or 14 jeans and wearing up to a 16 top – now I'm in 8–10 jeans and 10–12 tops. For me, it's not about the scales but how I feel in what I'm wearing and being comfortable in my own skin.'

And the health benefits have been even better than she expected: 'My psoriasis disappeared within weeks of starting fasting. I also used to get stress eczema flare-ups since the age of 21 – not any more. And how much better do you feel after fasting! There is certainly a feel-good factor to it, feeling more positive and cleansed.'

Karen's success persuaded her to tackle another health issue – giving up smoking. 'I stopped 10 months after I started 5:2. I believe that was a direct link to doing 5:2 and being more aware of my body. I wasn't a big smoker but kicking the few cigs I had made a big impact on my well-being.'

Fasting has also helped re-educate her diet. 'My attitude has definitely changed regarding food. Before 5:2 I didn't know very much about calories. Nowadays I tend to shop for a week's menu: this takes away all the hungry, grab-anything times. I want what I eat to be good for body and soul but still have a little indulgence and really appreciate it.'

Fast Day routine:

When I first started fasting I used to have lunch and dinner. Now I go all day without eating and have a small evening meal. Monday is usually a salad with an omelette or boiled eggs and Thursday is usually something quick and easy like a stir-fry or a rake about the fridge to use up veg in a soup. Mustn't forget the fasting friend the mushroom, how versatile is that! Fast Days are as normal as breathing now.

The other 5 days:

I try to have something for breakfast before work, then something like a Greek salad for lunch with a main meal at night. Weekends, I don't have any routine. Sometimes I will only eat once a day, others I graze when hungry, but we generally eat out a couple of times over the weekend. I don't calorie-count on any day now really. I have an idea on Fast Days but if I'm unsure I will do a quick cross-check on myfitnesspal.com – I believe my appetite is smaller now so I never overeat, I can't remember the last time I was bloated or uncomfortable after a meal.

The veggie life:

I work as a company secretary at a livestock mart, not exactly the perfect career for a veggie, but I've eaten this way for over thirty years. I never said I was turning vegetarian, I just stopped eating meat at an early age. Veggie food and 5:2 is a match made in heaven really, as you get lots of bulk for your calories on a Fast Day and it's nutritious, too, as long as you don't go adding lots of fat.

I love fresh, seasonal veg and what you can create in a short time.

Top tips:

It's OK, you will not die of starvation – a Fast Day is just one day. Always plan what you are going to eat on that day and check calorie counts. If it's easier to have a ready/calorie-counted meal, go for it, you will soon start cooking your own meals once you are into the way of things.

Last word:

I can't imagine not fasting now. You feel so good and virtuous after a fast, even after over three years of fasting. I do have breaks from fasting when I am on holiday but I get straight back on it when I return – it's just how I live my life now.

HERBY WILD MUSHROOM PARCEL, 155 Calories

(⊞)(✐)(✿) if gluten-free bread used

This is the perfect way to maximise the flavour of mushrooms, especially the more unusual varieties, such as shiitake, enoki and chanterelles. Their low calorie count means you can indulge in a little herb butter or oil when cooking them, and the parcels steam the fungi perfectly. The aroma when you open the parcel is to die for… I serve with sourdough bread I've sliced myself, as thinly as possible – it means you can still eat really good bread, if you enjoy it, but control the calories.

Serves 1
Preparation time: 5 minutes
Cooking time: 10 minutes

100g mixed wild or exotic mushrooms, sliced, around 25
    calories depending on variety
A few fresh herbs of your choice: chives, parsley, basil, 2
5g butter, 36, or 5ml extra-virgin olive oil, 41
Zest from ½ lemon, or a good pinch of chilli flakes, 2
Small slice of sourdough or gluten-free bread, around 40g, 90
Freshly ground sea salt and black pepper, to taste
Optional: Poached egg, 66 (see pages 77–79)

1. Preheat the oven to 200°C/400°F/Gas mark 6.

2. Cut or tear a dinner-plate-sized square of baking parchment or paper and place the mushrooms in the centre. Add the herbs, then the butter or oil and lemon zest or chilli. Season well. Fold the paper over the mushrooms

lengthways to enclose them, then scrunch the top and bottom ends to seal. Place the parcel on a baking tray and cook in the oven for around 10 minutes.

3. Toast the bread and place on plate, with more fresh herbs on the side.

4. Serve the unopened parcel next to the toast and egg (if using), so you get the full benefit of the delicious mushroom smell when you carefully open it up.

P.S. Experiment with different flavours: for example, coconut oil with a stalk of lemongrass gives these shrooms a Thai dimension. For a more substantial meal, serve with 50g avocado (80 calories) mashed and spread over the toast.

INDIAN CHILLI BREAKFAST PANCAKES, 120 calories per pancake

If you've never come across chickpea or 'gram' flour before, this is the recipe you should start with. Pancakes are commonly served for breakfast in many regions of India, and this is a glorious, golden, vegan and gluten-free version. Serve any time of day with your preferred accompaniment (see P.S. below).

Makes 4 pancakes
Preparation time: 10 minutes + resting for 1+ hours
Cooking time: 5–6 minutes per pancake

  1 small onion, 38
  1 green or red chilli, deseeded, 4
  100g gram flour, 336
  100ml warm water
  1 teaspoon garam masala, 5
  1 teaspoon turmeric, 5
  1 teaspoon whole spices of your choice – onion or mustard
      seeds, cumin seeds, 5
  ½ teaspoon sea salt (or to taste), 0
  ½ teaspoon baking powder, 3
  ½ teaspoon coconut or groundnut oil per pancake, 21, for
      frying

1. Finely chop the onion and chilli – it's fastest to do this in a food processor. Add the gram flour, water, spices, salt and baking powder and

blend again. Stir well, leave in a warm place overnight or for at least 1 hour until bubbles form.

2. Heat ½ teaspoon of oil in a small, non-stick frying pan (an omelette pan is ideal). When it's very hot, pour in around a quarter of the mix (about 65–75ml) and tilt the pan so the mix spreads across it. You can also use a spatula if the mix is very thick.

3. Turn the heat down and allow to cook for 2–3 minutes on one side, then carefully flip over and cook on the other side: it may take a little longer to cook now the temperature is lower, but make sure it's cooked right through. Serve immediately.

P. S. Make the batter in advance and keep in the fridge for up to 4–5 days to use when you wish. Shake or stir the batter well before using and fry as many pancakes as you need each time. Serve simply with a little yogurt and chutney or fresh herbs on top, or for a bigger meal, serve with fried or scrambled tofu or eggs (page 75 has a spicy version), with dal (page 106) or the Beany bunny, aka curry sandwich from page 136.

HOMEMADE BAKED BEANS ON TOAST, 195 calories

(🎁) (🥕) (🌾) if gluten-free bread used

Baked beans are comforting and nutritious, combining fibre-
and nutrient-rich beans with spices and tomato (which has
more available nutrients cooked than when raw). But rather
than opening a tin, why not try making your own with dried
cannellini beans? These beans are deliciously spicy and smoky,
served with a small slice of sourdough or wholegrain toast or as
part of a veggie full English.

Makes 4 servings
Preparation time: 5 minutes (plus soaking the beans overnight)
Cooking time: 1 hour 30 minutes

5g butter or coconut oil, 36–41
1 shallot, finely diced, 10
Pinch of freshly ground salt and pepper, 0
½ teaspoon ground cumin, 2.5
¼ teaspoon hot smoked paprika, 2
½ teaspoon celery salt, 2.5
1 level tablespoon tomato purée, 10–23
100g dried cannellini beans, 320, soaked overnight in cold
    water
1 teaspoon maple syrup, 13
100ml tomato passata, 25
4 x 40g slices of sourdough, wholemeal or gluten-free bread,
    around 90 each

1. Drain the soaked beans and rinse briefly. Gently heat the butter or oil in a saucepan and fry off the shallot for about 5 minutes until it begins to soften – add a pinch of salt as this helps stop the shallot burning, plus the pepper.

2. Add the spices to the pan and allow to cook out and coat the onions for a few minutes before adding the tomato purée and cooking for a two more minutes.

3. Add in the drained cannellini beans, maple syrup, passata and 300ml cold water. Bring to the boil and simmer for around 1 hour and 20 minutes, until the beans are tender and the sauce has thickened.

4. When you're ready, toast the bread and serve.

P. S. If you like things a little spicy, try adding more smoked paprika.

The beans keep well in the fridge for a few days or you can freeze them – but defrost them before reheating so the bean skins don't disintegrate on cooking.

AUSSIE SMOOTHIE WITH AVOCADO, KIWI AND PINK GRAPEFRUIT, 169 calories

Smoothies and juices can be useful for breakfast on the go, though I usually prefer to eat whole fruit or vegetables. This drink takes its inspiration from Australian produce, and the avocado here will keep you fuller for longer. It's not overly sweet, which I like, but you can add agave or honey if you want to tone down the tangy grapefruit.

Serves 1
Preparation time: 5 minutes

> ½ small avocado, around 50g flesh cut into chunks, 80
> 1 kiwi, peeled, one slice reserved, 42
> ½ small pink grapefruit, peeled, one slice reserved, 25
> 20g or a good handful of spinach, 5
> 150ml almond milk, 17
> Pinch of sea salt
> *Optional: ½ teaspoon agave nectar or honey, 8–10*

1. Add the avocado, kiwi and grapefruit to a blender with the other ingredients and blend until smooth.

2. Garnish with a slice of kiwi or grapefruit. If you're making it to drink later, then keep in the fridge until needed.

P. S. Alternatively, you can serve this as a salad rather than a smoothie: slice the fruit, dice the avocado and use the juice from the other half of the grapefruit as a dressing.

BAKED AVOCADO STUFFED WITH BEANS AND SMOKED CHEESE, 209 calories

This is one of my favourite dishes of all time: eating a version of this when I was 18, way before avocados were trendy, made me realise how exciting veggie food could be. The flavour of avocados becomes nuttier and richer when they are gently baked. I've added beans here (you don't need many, use whatever you have), paprika and smoked cheese. One tip: use very fresh avocados, as an older one becomes stringy when baked.

Serves 1
Preparation time: 8 minutes
Cooking time: 10–12 minutes

½ small avocado, 100–120 calories depending on size
30g cooked, drained beans, such as borlotti, 28
¼ teaspoon paprika, 3
1 spring onion, finely sliced, 2
10g smoked cheese, 38
Freshly ground sea salt and black pepper, to taste

To serve

1 dessertspoon half-fat crème fraiche, 18,
5 cherry tomatoes, 15–25
2 small wedges cut from an iceberg lettuce, 5

1. Preheat the oven to 180°C/350°F/Gas mark 4.

2. Cut the avocado in half and remove the stone. Lightly crush the beans with the paprika and mix with the sliced spring onion.

3. Place the avocado on a baking tray and pile the bean mix into its centre, to cover. Slice the cheese *very* thinly to cover the beans and as much flesh as possible. Bake in the oven for 10–12 minutes.

4. Season and serve with the crème fraiche, plus the cherry tomatoes and lettuce wedges – these are great for scooping up the hot filling.

P. S. The same technique works well with cream cheese or a blue cheese like Stilton, with a topping of walnuts on a non-Fast Day. For a vegan version, top the beans with mixed seeds and a good sprinkling of nutritional yeast.

SPICED BRUNCH SCRAMBLE, 159–176 calories

Vegan option with tofu: 159
Veggie option with egg: 176

Quick, easy, filling – what more could you want from a breakfast dish? Though actually, I like this as a TV dinner, too, with a pitta bread or small chapatti.

Serves 1
Preparation time: 4 minutes
Cooking time: 4–8 minutes

100g firm plain tofu, 115, or 2 medium eggs, 132
½ teaspoon coconut or groundnut/rapeseed oil, 21
1 teaspoon garam masala, 5
½ teaspoon mustard seeds or nigella/onion seeds, 3
3 cherry tomatoes, finely chopped, 9–15
1 small red or green chilli pepper, deseeded and finely
    chopped, 4
1 small spring onion, finely chopped, 2
Freshly ground sea salt and black pepper, to taste
Optional: coriander sprigs, to garnish

1. If using eggs, break them into a mug and beat lightly with a fork. For the tofu, drain from the packet and use kitchen roll to press out as much moisture as you can. Break up with a fork.

2. Heat the oil in a small non-stick saucepan. Add the spices, chilli, spring onion and tomatoes, and fry over a high heat for 2 minutes. Now lower the heat and add the eggs or tofu. For the eggs, move them around the pan as the egg sets, until they reach the texture you like (remember they carry on cooking once you've turned off the heat). For the tofu, sauté until the edges are lightly browned.

3. Serve on a warm plate, season with salt and pepper and garnish, if you like, with coriander leaves.

P. S. Add a chopped garlic clove to the pan at Step 2, taking care not to burn it. Serve with a small chapatti or the Indian pancake from page 76. For a Mexican flavour, use ground cumin and dried thyme instead of the garam masala and mustard/onion seeds.

PEA AND HERB PANCAKES WITH WATERCRESS AND POACHED EGGS, 222 calories

There's so much to love about these: they look gorgeous on the plate and they taste delicate and sophisticated. They're also made mostly from freezer and storecupboard ingredients. The perfect brunch or supper for two: or for cooking two days running – just keep the batter covered in the fridge and give it a quick mix before using.

Serves 2
Preparation time: 10 minutes
Cooking time: 9–10 minutes
Pancakes 127 calories per serving

> 150g frozen peas, 90
> Good bunch/10g chopped herbs, such as dill, mint or chives, 5
> 1 egg, 66
> 1 tablespoon cornflour, 57
> 5g butter, 36, or 5ml oil, 41
> Freshly ground sea salt and black pepper, to taste

For the topping, 95 per serving
> Splash of vinegar
> 2 eggs, 132
> 20g watercress, 5
> 2 level tablespoons half-fat crème fraiche, 52

1. Cook the peas in a pan of boiling water or in the microwave according to the packet instructions. Meanwhile, bring some water to the boil in a medium saucepan to poach the eggs for topping the dish.

2. Blend the cooked peas and chopped herbs using a hand blender, reserving a few herb leaves for garnish. Add the egg and cornflour and blend until well mixed. Season well.

3. Heat the butter or oil in a large non-stick frying pan, and when hot, make 4 pancakes by spooning 2 level tablespoons of the pea batter **per pancake** into onto the pan, keeping the pancakes separate (if you don't have a large enough pan, do this in two batches, keeping the first set warm on a plate in a low oven while you cook the others).

4. Cook over a high heat for 2–3 minutes until the bottoms are lightly browned and the tops are set enough to turn. Turn carefully using a spatula and knife and lower the temperature, then cook for another 2–3 minutes.

5. Meanwhile, poach the eggs: add a splash of vinegar to the pan with the boiling water. Break the first egg into a cup. Create a whirlpool in the water with a fork or whisk and, with your other hand, slip the egg into the middle of the saucepan as gently as possible. Repeat with the second egg. Turn off the heat and set a timer for 3 minutes. After that time, check that the egg whites have set before removing from the saucepan using a slotted spoon. Place onto a plate lined with kitchen roll to absorb the excess cooking water.

6. Arrange the watercress on one side of a plate and place two pancakes alongside. Place the poached egg on top of the pancakes and spoon the crème fraiche next to it, topped with the reserved herb leaves. Season and serve immediately.

P. S. The pancakes are delicious with a little mustard powder added to the mixture, or with French mustard on the side. They also go well with other breakfast items such as fried mushrooms or veggie sausages: serve with baby spinach rather than watercress if you prefer.

FRESH CORN AND BLACK BEAN TACOS, 247 calories

Vegan with seeds: 247 per serving
Vegetarian with crème fraiche: 258 per serving

This is so colourful and delicious, a fantastic sharing dish for brunch for two (my partner said: 'I'd pay good money for this in our local Mexican restaurant.'). The black beans and salsa keep well in the fridge, so if you're eating alone, you can eat this two days running. You can use shop-bought salsa if you're in a rush, and to make it even faster, simply use frozen or tinned corn instead of a fresh corn on the cob.

Serves 2
Preparation time: 5 minutes
Cooking time: 10 minutes

100g sweetcorn from 1 medium 180g corn on the cob, or 100g frozen/tinned corn, 90

1 heaped tablespoon tomato salsa (shop-bought, or see recipe page 138), 10–20

½ tin black beans, 120g, drained, 108

½ teaspoon dried oregano, 3

½ teaspoon chilli flakes, 3

Juice of 1 lime, 12

2 corn tortillas, 222 (sizes vary so check packaging)

For the topping, 45–67 per serving

30g or 2 good handfuls shredded lettuce, 5
4 radishes, sliced, 4
Jalapeño peppers from a jar, to taste, sliced, 6 per pepper
2 level tablespoons half-fat crème fraiche, 52 or 1 teaspoon
    pumpkin and sesame seeds, 30

1. Heat a griddle and cook the corn on the cob for 8–10 minutes, turning often so the kernels turn golden brown. When cooled, run a sharp knife down the cob to remove the kernels. If using frozen, cook them following the instructions. Mix with the salsa.

2. Meanwhile, heat the black beans in a small pan with the oregano, chilli flakes and lime juice, lightly mashing the beans with the spatula or a fork.

3. When you're ready to serve, heat the tortillas on the griddle until crispy. Spread the base with the black beans, pile on the corn salsa, some of the lettuce, sliced radishes and jalapeños. Add the crème fraiche or seeds and serve with more lettuce on the side.

P. S. If you're following a gluten-free diet, check your tortillas are made with no wheat as some use a mix of corn and wheat flour. On a non-Fast Day, this is delicious with sliced avocado or a good grating of Cheddar cheese.

YOGURT-BAKED TRUFFLED EGGS WITH GREEN LEAVES, 247 calories

This is indulgent and rich, and excellent 'calorie value' – serve with a good handful of rocket leaves to cut through the richness of the eggs. The water bath or bain marie helps prevent the egg mix splitting or going watery, as does using full-fat yogurt.

Serves 1
Preparation time: 5 minutes
Cooking time: 18–22 minutes

70ml full-fat Greek yogurt, 67
2 medium eggs, 132
½ teaspoon truffle oil or extra-virgin olive oil, 21
A few fresh herb leaves, such as chives or tarragon, 1
5g Grana Padano, 20, or vegetarian Gruyère cheese, 25
Freshly ground sea salt and black pepper, to taste
20g rocket leaves or watercress, 6, to serve

1. Preheat the oven to 150°C/300°F/Gas mark 2, and boil some water in a kettle.

2. Spoon just over half the yogurt into the bottom of a small, shallow, ovenproof dish. Carefully break the eggs and place on top of the yogurt. Add the oil and fresh herbs, then spoon the rest of the yogurt on the top. Season well, then grate the cheese over the top.

3. Place the dish into a larger ovenproof dish or roasting tin and carefully fill the larger container with enough boiling water to reach a centimetre or so below the edge of the smaller dish: make sure the water doesn't splash into the egg mix.

4. Bake for 18–22 minutes, depending on how you like your eggs: at 18 minutes, the yolks will still be runny, firmer after 22 minutes. Serve in the dish, with watercress or rocket on the side.

P. S. Try serving with roast balsamic tomatoes: perfect if you have some leftover cherry tomatoes that are going wrinkly. Place 10 cherry tomatoes, 30–50 calories depending on size, in a small roasting dish; season well and add a tablespoon of balsamic vinegar, 5–20. Roast at the same time as the eggs.

CINNAMON BUCKWHEAT PORRIDGE WITH FIG AND STRAWBERRIES, 245 calories

Buckwheat porridge is fashionable right now, for good reason – it's filling, tasty and gluten-free. The toasted flavour of the buckwheat compliments the warming maple syrup and cinnamon sweetness. The fig and strawberry compote makes a great topping – prepare four portions on Sunday to speed up weekday breakfasts!

Serves 1
Preparation time: 5 minutes
Cooking time: 15 minutes

    100ml nut milk, such as almond, 13
    100ml water, 0
    45g toasted buckwheat, 170
    ½ teaspoon ground cinnamon, 3
    Pinch of sea salt, 0
    1 tablespoon maple syrup, 40

For the poached fruit compote, makes 4 portions, 19 per serving

    1 small fresh fig, quartered, 43
    100g strawberries, hulled and quartered, 32
    A sprinkling of ground cinnamon, to dust, 0

1. Put the milk and water in a medium saucepan and add the buckwheat, reserving 1 dessertspoonful. Heat gently until just below boiling. Turn the heat down to low.

2. Add the cinnamon, salt and maple syrup and simmer for 5 minutes. Add the reserved buckwheat and cook for a further 10 minutes.

3. To make the compote, gently cook the fig and strawberries in a splash of water in a separate pan until soft and releasing their juices. Keep covered in the fridge.

4. Serve the porridge with a dessertspoon of the compote and an extra dusting of cinnamon.

P. S. If you can't find figs, just substitute another berry – blueberries or blackberries – and adjust the calories.

CHAPTER TWO

Soup

Soup is a Fast Day lifesaver. It's cheap, portable, delicious – and it keeps us fuller for longer. From wintry soups that fuel you all day long to a light, summery tomato broth or a deep, turmeric-scented dish of Indian dal, this chapter is packed with ideas to soup up your mealtimes.

RECIPES

VIETNAMESE SPICY PHO WITH FRESH HERBS AND COURGETTE NOODLES, ⓥ ✓ 🌾, 70

SUPER-GREEN BROCCOLI SOUP WITH AN UMAMI KICK, ⓥ ✓ 🌾, 73

FRAGRANT TOMATO BROTH WITH FRESH HERBS, ⓥ ✓ 🌾, 97

HIKER'S HEARTY BEAN AND LEEK SOUP WITH HOT PAPRIKA, ⓥ ✓ 🌾, 121

SMOKED CHILLI VELVET SOUP, ⓥ ✓ 🌾, 126
(or 91 with butternut squash)

CHICKPEA AND WILD MUSHROOM WARMER, ⓥ ✓ 🌾, 142

MUSHROOM AND MANGETOUT SOUP WITH MISO NOODLES, ⓥ ✓ 🌾, 146

COMFORTING LENTIL DAL WITH FRIED SPICY ONIONS, ⓥ ✓ 🌾, 280

HOMEMADE VEGGIE STOCK ⓥ ✓ 🌾, 24

5:2 Lives

JO AND JAN'S FASTING JOURNEY TO ZANZIBAR

'It's very easy because we approach it as a lifestyle change and not a diet.'

Before: 1 stone (15kg) heavier thanks to a shared love of good food
After: back in a bikini and still cooking together

For Jo Charnock, 47, and her partner Jan, living together and cooking together was a shared passion – but it came at a price.

'Since I met Jan, 13 years ago, I steadily picked up weight as we both enjoy cooking and good food. I used to joke that he was a 'feeder'. The last couple of years, I really started to feel 'fat'; I was about a stone (15kg) heavier than when we met. My partner had no problem with it but I just didn't feel good any more. But I don't believe in diets, as when you stop the diet, what's to stop the weight piling back on.'

It's a problem most dieters have encountered. So Jo decided to look beyond the traditional calorie-counting regimes. 'A friend of mine did a 21-day water diet for cleansing and spiritual reasons. I couldn't believe that someone could function normally on just water for 21 days. She sent me some info to read about the different types of fasting, and with a bit more research I came across the 5:2 diet, which made more sense to me. I also spend a lot of time living in a Muslim country, so I'm familiar with the Ramadan fast. Having a regular fasting time just made sense to me.'

Jan was equally keen to do the 5:2. 'There was no real preparation, but we were going to do it together, which helps. We just decided to start on a Monday. I was fine, but my partner felt cold and a little feverish the first day, but we've both been fine since then. It's very easy as we approach it as a lifestyle change and not a diet.'

That lifestyle change came while they were working in Zanzibar, building two bungalows to rent out and running bicycle tours. But they didn't have a bathroom scale out there, so Jo had to wait to weigh herself until she got home to Cape Town, South Africa.

'I've lost 8kg in three months and have gone from a size 12–14 back to a 10. Most of my clothes are too big for me now. I have even been in public in a bikini!'

Fast Day routine:

I only have black tea and water on a fasting day, so no food. Hunger pangs come and go in the afternoon. Instead of cooking, we normally end up in bed early with a movie. Our friends also know not to bother us to go out on fasting days . . .

The other 5 days:

On non-fasting days we eat a varied diet; we both love Italian food, so there is quite a lot of pasta involved. In Zanzibar, you are quite limited with what is available and it's very seasonal, too, so you have to be creative. We both love spicy food, and we grow our own chillies in the garden. Now we're back in Cape Town for a month and it's asparagus season, so we're spoiling ourselves with all kinds of different dishes! There's no calorie-counting, or routine change, just eating smaller portions.

The veggie life:

I have been vegetarian for about 32 years, mainly for ethical reasons. I am not against people eating meat per se, but I am against factory farming and people being completely unaware of where their meat comes from or the conditions in which animals are kept. Veggie eating is definitely more creative, and people always comment about how good our food is.

Top tips:

Try to stick to regular Fast days, and if it doesn't always work, don't be too hard on yourself.

Last word:

So far, it really has become part of our weekly routine, and we both actually look forward to our fasting days. 5:2 doesn't always work out with our social life, but we always manage at least one day per week, which helps maintain the weight loss. I'm definitely more aware of how much I'm eating, and I stop when I'm full instead of always trying to finish my plate.

VIETNAMESE SPICY PHO WITH FRESH HERBS AND COURGETTE NOODLES, 70 calories

OK, this has a long list of ingredients, but it's so fresh, light and spicy, and packs lots of vegetables into one uplifting bowl. The method is simple, too: make the broth, briefly cook the veg, then tuck in. The courgettes are prepared like 'courgetti' (see page 213) and I use a small, inexpensive julienne peeler rather than a spiraliser – much less washing up, though do watch your fingers! You can make several batches of the broth in advance and freeze or keep in a container in the fridge to reduce the cooking time. You can make this with courgette noodles (which I prefer, it's so light) or rice noodles.

NB: The calories listed here don't include the aromatics added to the soup, because they're removed before you eat it.

Serves 1
Preparation time: 10 minutes
Cooking time: 15 minutes

For the broth (see note in the introduction)

    1 garlic clove, sliced
    ½ red chilli, sliced (leave out if you prefer a milder flavour)
    1cm piece of fresh ginger, peeled and sliced
    1 lemongrass stalk, cut in half and lightly crushed
    ½ onion, cut in half
    1 star anise or 2 cloves (you can reuse after drying out)

For the vegetables

30g exotic mushrooms, sliced, 8

30g mangetout or green beans, 10

30g pak choi, leaves separated, 4

30g carrot, sliced into matchsticks, 9

Zest and juice of ½ lime, 8

75g courgette, cut into noodles with a julienne peeler or
   spiraliser (see above), 13

In the bowl

Small handful mixed herbs: coriander, Thai basil and mint, 5

½ red chilli, finely sliced, 2

25g beansprouts from a tin, rinsed, or fresh, 8 (see safety note
   below)

1 spring onion, chopped, 3

*Optional: 3g peanuts, lightly crushed, 18 (calorie count with
   nuts, 91), to garnish*

1. Place all the broth ingredients in a saucepan with 400ml water. Bring to
   boil and simmer for 10 minutes.

2. Meanwhile, lightly chop the herbs for the bowl and place half in your
   serving bowl, along with the chilli, plus the beansprouts if using tinned.

3. Strain the broth through a sieve, discarding the aromatics (or you
   can reuse in another soup). Return the broth to the pan, add all the
   vegetables, the fresh beansprouts, if using, (they need to be cooked well)
   and lime juice. Bring to boil then reduce to a simmer for 2 minutes. Add
   the courgette noodles and simmer for another 2 minutes.

4. Pour the hot soup and vegetables over the herbs. Top with the chopped spring onion, the remaining herbs, lime zest and the crushed peanuts, if using, and serve immediately.

Important: Handle fresh beansprouts carefully as, surprisingly, they are a very common cause of food poisoning. Rinse well and discard if smelly, brown or even slightly musty. If you are immune-compromised or are serving this to children, the elderly or pregnant women, simmer for at least 4 minutes before serving, or use shredded lettuce instead. Canned beansprouts can be safer and taste pretty good.

P. S. For a slightly higher-calorie version with rice noodles, replace the courgetti with 25g/around half a nest of thick no-cook rice noodles (92 calories). Prepare according to the packet instructions, then place in the bottom of the bowl along with the herbs and pour the soup over. It increases the calorie count to 149.

SUPER-GREEN BROCCOLI SOUP WITH AN UMAMI KICK, 73 calories

Vegan version: with oil and nutritional yeast, 73
Veggie version: with butter and blue cheese, 83

This is a *really* simple soup but it's super-delicious. The secret? Nutritional yeast – aka 'nooch' – that gives it the savoury 'umami' flavour that chefs love. If you like broccoli and Stilton soup, you'll enjoy this too. If you're veggie rather than vegan, you can also add blue cheese when serving for an umami double-whammy…

Serves 4
Preparation time: 5 minutes
Cooking time: 12 minutes

1 onion, chopped, 38
2 garlic cloves, chopped, 8
1 teaspoon butter, 36, or rapeseed/groundnut oil, 41
400g broccoli florets, 128
600ml veggie stock (see page 108) or made with 2 teaspoons of vegetable bouillon, 24
1 teaspoon nutritional yeast, 17
Freshly ground sea salt and black pepper, to taste
10g nutritional yeast, 34, or 25g blue cheese, crumbled, 81, to serve

1. Fry the onion and garlic with the butter or oil in a large saucepan for 2 minutes.

2. Add the broccoli florets to the pan with the stock and nutritional yeast. Bring to the boil and let the broccoli cook for 8–10 minutes until tender but not mushy.

3. Blend in the pan to a creamy consistency: if you like a thinner soup, add water, 100ml at a time. Season well.

4. Sprinkle the yeast or blue cheese evenly among the 4 bowls, or use a quarter each time if serving on different days.

P. S. Broccoli and chilli go so well together, so add either 1 chopped chilli or a teaspoon of dried chilli flakes (or more/less to taste) at step 1.

This soup freezes well: just add the cheese or yeast toppings after thawing and reheating.

FRAGRANT TOMATO BROTH WITH FRESH HERBS, 97 calories

This special soup tastes of an Italian summer: ripe tomatoes, fresh herbs and olive oil. It's perfect to make if your homegrown crop has gone crazy (they are easy to grow even in a small space) or the supermarket or local veg stall is selling off seasonal ripe tomatoes at rock-bottom prices.

The broth looks beautiful – it is almost transparent, with an intense hit of tomato flavour and delicate green herbs floating on the top.

Serves 2
Preparation time: 25 minutes
Cooking time: 5 minutes

> 1.5kg ripe tomatoes (270 calories BUT only around half of
>   calories used in the soup), roughly chopped, 135
> 2 shallots, peeled and roughly chopped, 4
> Juice of 1 lemon, 12
> Handful of basil leaves, 5
> Handful of parsley leaves, 5
> Freshly ground sea salt and black pepper, to taste

For the vegetable garnish, 16.5 per serving

> 1 medium ripe tomato, 15
> ½ small courgette, 17
> 1 dill sprig, 1
> *Optional dressing: 1 teaspoon extra-virgin olive oil or basil oil,*
>   *41 (adds 21 cals per person)*

1. Place the tomatoes and shallots in a food processor along with the lemon juice, salt, pepper, basil and parsley, reserving a few leaves for the garnish, and blitz to a pulp. You can also use a hand blender.

2. Line a fine sieve with a cheesecloth or clean J-cloth and place over a large bowl. Tip in the tomato pulp and leave to sit for about 15 minutes – you can stir the pulp occasionally and push down lightly with a spoon to get as much juice out as possible.

3. While the mixture is straining, prepare the vegetable garnish. Quarter the tomato and remove the centre. Finely dice the flesh and divide among 2 serving bowls. Do the same with the courgette. Then snip the dill and sprinkle on top of the vegetables.

4. The tomato juice in the bottom of the bowl should now be clear and golden. Heat gently in a saucepan over a low heat until just below boiling, then pour over the prepared vegetables in the 2 bowls. (Don't discard the pulp, though – see P.S. for ideas as to what you can do with it.)

5. Finally, garnish with a few drops of oil, if using.

P. S. The second portion will keep, covered, in the fridge for up to three days – so will any leftover tomato pulp (it's not got much flavour, but works well in another soup or in a lentil spaghetti Bolognese on a non-Fast Day).

HIKER'S HEARTY BEAN AND LEEK SOUP WITH HOT PAPRIKA, 121 calories

I always imagine tucking into this after a hike across in a chilly, bright forest (though it works just as well after a long day at work!). It has a Hungarian feel which comes from the use of paprika. If using dried beans, soak them overnight to reduce the cooking time. I like to add a little extra paprika or hot pepper sauce when serving.

Serves 4, 121 calories
Preparation time: 15 minutes
Cooking time: 20–25 minutes (1 hour if using dried beans)

- 1 x 400g tin cannellini beans, drained, or 75g dried cannellini beans, 238–250
- 150g carrots, diced, 51
- 1 medium celery stick, diced, 60g, 6
- 2 medium leeks, diced,200g, 112
- 5g butter, 36, or 1 teaspoon rapeseed/groundnut oil, 41
- 1 bay leaf, 0
- 5 rosemary sprigs, chopped, or 1 teaspoon dried, 5
- 5 thyme sprigs, or 1 teaspoon dried, 5
- 900ml vegetable stock made from 2 teaspoons vegetable bouillon or homemade, around 24
- 1 teaspoon paprika, 5
- *Optional: a few drops of hot pepper sauce in each bowl, 1 or less*

1. If using dried beans, soak them in cold water overnight. Rinse and drain the next morning.

2. Heat the butter/oil in a large saucepan and gently fry the carrots, celery and leeks for 5 minutes. Add the bay leaf, chopped rosemary and the thyme leaves (reserve a few for garnish if using fresh), followed by the beans and the stock.

3. Bring to a simmer. If using tinned beans, cook until the carrot has softened, around 20 minutes. If using dried beans, simmer for up to 1 hour until the beans are cooked through: stir regularly and add more water if required.

4. If you like a smooth soup, use a stick blender to blend once the beans are cooked.

5. Season and serve, with the reserved herbs, a little sprinkle of paprika, or a few drops of hot chilli sauce stirred through, if you like.

P. S. Use any combination of beans and vegetables: 50g quick-cook farro (emmer wheat, 181 calories, not gluten-free) added to the soup 12 minutes before the end of cooking will make it even heartier.

SMOKED CHILLI VELVET SOUP, 126 calories
(91 made with butternut squash)

This is a velvety, creamy soup with a kick of smoked chilli – truly warming for a winter's day, and completely vegan-friendly, as the creamy texture comes from white beans. The sweet potatoes make for a creamier soup, while the squash gives a much lower-cal result. Buy dried chipotles or chipotle paste in larger supermarkets – or Amazon stock them. They're quite strong, so use less if you prefer a mellow soup. Alternatively, use a fat fresh chilli with a teaspoon of smoked paprika. This freezes like a dream!

Serves 4
Preparation time: 10 minutes
Cooking time: 25–30 minutes

- 1 dried chipotle pepper, 23, or chipotle paste, to taste (1 teaspoon is around 8 cals)
- 5g butter or coconut oil, 36–41
- 300g sweet potatoes (1 large), 258, or butternut squash, peeled and cut into cubes, 120
- 1 small onion, chopped, 38
- 1 teaspoon whole cumin seeds, 5
- 1 litre vegetable stock, homemade, or with 2 teaspoons vegetable bouillon, 24
- ½ x 400g tin cooked cannellini beans, drained, 119

Optional topping: 1 level tablespoon half-fat crème fraiche, 26, or coconut yogurt, 8–29 per bowl

1. Rehydrate the dried chipotle, if using, in a small dish of hot water for a few minutes. Remove the seeds from the inside of the chipotle with a knife (unless you like a very strong chilli flavour) and chop roughly.

2. Gently heat the butter or oil in a large saucepan and fry the sweet potatoes (or butternut squash), onion, chipotle or chipotle paste and whole cumin seeds for 5 minutes. Add the stock and beans, bring to a simmer and cook for 20–25 minutes, until the potatoes or squash are soft.

3. Blend to a very smooth texture. Serve with the crème fraiche or yogurt swirled in, if using.

P. S. You can replace the cannellini beans with any other pulse – black beans would be a good fit for the Mexican spicing.

CHICKPEA AND WILD MUSHROOM WARMER, 142 calories (162–163 with topping)

This Italian-influenced soup has a deeply savoury flavour. As a kid, before I went veggie, we'd have hot oxtail soup to warm us up – and this has the same soothing, satisfying depth, without the meat! It's a great winter meal because mushrooms are rich in myconutrients, which boost the immune system without increasing inflammation. For this dish dried mushroom pieces are fine, as they're better value than the whole ones: truffle oil is optional but it does add extra glamour.

Serves 4
Preparation time: 8 minutes
Cooking time: 12 minutes

10g dried wild or porcini mushrooms, 25
5g butter, 36, or 1 teaspoon rapeseed/groundnut oil, 41
2 garlic cloves, chopped or crushed, 8
1 onion, sliced, 38
Handful of herb leaves, such as rosemary, oregano or
    1 teaspoon dried Italian herbs, 5
300g chestnut mushrooms, roughly chopped, 66
1 x 400g tin chickpeas, drained, 312
250ml passata, 64
500ml vegetable stock, made with water and 1 teaspoon
    vegetable bouillon, 12
Freshly ground sea salt and black pepper, to taste

*Optional: 5g grated Grana Padano cheese per serving, 20, or
½ teaspoon truffle/basil oil, 21*

1. Rehydrate the dried mushrooms in a bowl with around 75ml of hot water for a few minutes.

2. Melt the butter or oil in a large saucepan, then gently fry the garlic, onion and herbs for 3 minutes, before adding the fresh mushrooms and chickpeas and frying for 3 more minutes.

3. Add the dried mushrooms with their soaking liquid, the passata and the stock. Bring to a simmer and cook for 5 minutes.

4. Blend the soup in the pan with a stick blender: warm up again, season, and serve with a few fresh rosemary leaves, plus the cheese or oil, if using.

P. S. You can use cannellini or borlotti beans in place of the chickpeas, or add 100g baby spinach (25 calories) at step 4 and blend as before.

MUSHROOM AND MANGETOUT SOUP WITH MISO NOODLES, 146 calories

(ⓘ) (✎) (🌾) (if using gluten-free noodles, such as 100% buckwheat)

Brilliant green mangetout look glorious in this filling yet elegant soup, floating next to exotic mushrooms and noodles in a dark, savoury, miso-scented broth. You can use the milder shiro miso or the more savoury brown rice version – taste as you go to get the perfect flavour for you. Neither the seaweed nor the dried mushrooms are essential but they both give the broth a richer flavour.

Serves 1
Preparation time: 5 minutes
Cooking time: 10 minutes

25g udon or soba noodles, 86

300ml water

1 teaspoon soy or tamari sauce, 3–10

1cm piece of fresh ginger, peeled and grated, 2

1 garlic clove, grated, 4

1 medium spring onion, white parts chopped, green parts finely sliced, 2

2–3 dried shiitake mushrooms, 6

40g mixed mushrooms, 10–15

60g pak choi (1 baby pak choi or several larger leaves), 9–12

40g mangetout, 13

1–2 teaspoons miso paste (depending on the miso), 8–20

Optional: good pinch of dried mixed seaweed flakes, e.g. nori, dulse, wakame, 3, to serve

1. Cook the noodles according to instructions – they usually take less than 10 minutes. Rinse off after cooking.

2. While the noodles are cooking, prepare the broth. Bring the water to the boil in a small saucepan and add the soy or tamari, grated ginger and garlic, white parts of the spring onion and dried mushrooms. Bring to a simmer.

3. About 3 minutes before the noodles are ready, add the fresh mushrooms, pak choi and mangetout to the hot broth as it simmers. Place the miso paste in a small bowl, ladle over a little of the hot broth and whisk together: you don't want to boil the miso as it changes the flavour.

4. To serve, add the cooked noodles to the simmering broth and vegetables, pour into a serving dish and then mix in the diluted miso. Top with the green sliced spring onions and the seaweed flakes if using.

P. S. For a more substantial dish, add 75g smoked tofu (around 85 calories: check label) at step 2. You can vary the vegetables according to what you have: thinly sliced carrot or baby sweetcorn look so colourful but need a little longer to cook at step 3.

COMFORTING LENTIL DAL WITH FRIED SPICY ONIONS, 280 calories

Is it a soup? Is it a curry? You can enjoy it as both! In India, dal means both the many different pulses you cook with and also countless lentil-based soups and curries. The dish has two parts: the cooked lentils themselves, which are incredibly comforting on their own, and the spicy fried onion dressing or 'tarka'.

Makes 4 servings (or 8 side dish portions)
Preparation time: 5 minutes
Cooking time: 25–30 minutes

For the dal, 243 per portion (or 118 as a side dish)

    250g red split lentils, 883
    1 small onion, chopped, 38
    1 small red chilli, chopped, 4
    2cm piece of fresh ginger, peeled and grated, 4
    1 teaspoon turmeric, 5
    100g tomatoes, roughly chopped, 18
    75g spinach, 19
    Freshly ground sea salt and black pepper, to taste

For the tarka (fried spicy onions): serves 4, 37 calories per person

    1 teaspoon whole cumin and mustard seeds, 8
    15g butter, 108, or 3 teaspoons coconut oil, 123

½ small onion, thinly sliced, 19
2 garlic cloves, thinly sliced, 8
1 red chilli, deseeded and finely sliced, 4

1. Rinse the red lentils well and place in a saucepan with the onion, chilli, ginger, turmeric, chopped tomatoes and 1 litre of water. Bring to the boil then simmer for 20–25 minutes until the texture is between a soup and a purée. Skim off any foam that appears on the top.

2. While the lentils are cooking, wash the spinach, and remove any tough stalks. When the lentils are cooked, add the spinach and heat through. Season well and thin out with a little water if you want a thinner soup.

3. Meanwhile, toast the cumin and mustard seeds in a dry, non-stick frying pan until the seeds begin to pop. Add the butter or oil and sliced onion and fry until the onion is crisping up, 3–4 minutes.

4. Turn down the heat and add the garlic and chilli and fry until gently browned. To serve, add a little of the spiced onion to the top of each bowl of hot dal.

P. S. This dal is brilliant served with the pancakes on page 68, with cauliflower rice from page 202, or taken to work in a flask as a hot soup. Experiment with different lentils, following the packet instructions as most types take a little longer to cook than split red lentils. You can also vary your tarka – add different whole spices, garam masala, curry leaves, shallots or ginger. For a more indulgent dal – wonderful on a non-fasting day – use a little less water to cook and add 100ml coconut milk (233 calories) towards the end of the cooking time.

HOMEMADE VEGGIE/VEGAN STOCK, around 24 calories per 500ml

I don't *always* make homemade stock, often I use a bouillon powder like Marigold, which I think gives a natural-tasting soup base. But making stock is so easy and I like to get a pot bubbling away when I have lots of leftover pieces of veggie stalks or peel.

In veggie stock you can choose how much fat you use, though it's hard to estimate exactly how many calories the stock contains as the bulky ingredients are strained off. If you are using the stock as a base for Asian soups and stews, try using the same amount of coconut oil.

Makes 500ml (enough for 1 batch of soup)
Preparation time: 3 minutes
Cooking time: 18–23 minutes
Approx. 24 calories per portion

½ teaspoon rapeseed/groundnut oil
2 onions or leeks, chopped roughly, or the trimmings from other
    recipes
2 carrots, chopped into chunks (don't bother to peel), or
    trimmings
1 celery stick, chopped into chunks
Other vegetable trimmings/skins/ends: mushrooms stalks,
    tomato skin, parsnip ends, the ends of garlic, fennel
Herbs/spices: a bay leaf, ½ teaspoon peppercorns, sprig of
    thyme, some woodier parsley stems, chilli flakes

1. Heat the rapeseed/groundnut oil in a large saucepan.

2. Fry all the veg and herbs/spices until they're lightly browned and you can smell some of their flavour releasing.

3. Add 500–600ml water, bring to the boil, then simmer for 15–20 minutes. Turn off the heat and leave the vegetables in the cooling water for as long as possible before straining through a sieve. Allow to cool.

4. The liquid will keep for several days in the fridge, or freeze soup-sized portions for up to a year – you can melt them straight into the pan.

P. S. I often freeze my stock in an ice-cube tray before removing the cubes and storing in a plastic box/freezer bag. You could also keep a stock bag/tub in the fridge or freezer, and add trimmings to it as you have them until you have enough to make a stock (check nothing's gone mouldy first).

CHAPTER THREE

Lunchbox

Say goodbye to depressing canteen stodge or shrink-wrapped sandwiches. This chapter is about making lunch on the go something you'll look forward to all morning – and a meal your colleagues will envy. These dishes are also brilliant for a picnic; or if you work shifts, you could enjoy them as a midnight feast...

RECIPES

ARTICHOKE PÂTÉ WITH GRILLED RED CHICORY, ⑦⑦⑦, 58

ROCKET AND RICOTTA FRITTATA MUFFINS, ⑦⑦, 79

MINTY BEETROOT CAVIAR WITH RAINBOW CRUDITÉS, ⑦⑦⑦,113

CHESTNUT, LEEK AND MUSHROOM 'SAUSAGE' ROLLS, ⑦⑦, 144

SUPER-SAVOURY MISO AUBERGINE, ⑦⑦⑦,163

PACKED LUNCH PEPPER AND KALE MISO NOODLES, ⑦⑦⑦, 247

ONION BHAJI LUNCHBOX OMELETTE, ⑦⑦, 179

MUSHROOM AND CHILLI JAM QUESADILLA, ⑦⑦, 213, with pop-art coleslaw, 52

PEACAMOLE MINT TOSTADAS WITH RED PEPPER, ⑦⑦⑦, 218

PUY LENTIL STUFFED RAMIRO PEPPERS, ⑦⑦option⑦, 258 with lime pickled onions, 26

BEANY BUNNY, AKA CURRY SANDWICH, ⑦⑦, 268

SALSAS, ⑦⑦⑦, 20–50

5:2 Lives

JACKY'S FRENCH-STYLE 5:2
(with wine and cheese, oh la la!)

'A way of life, rather than just a diet...'

Before: stuck in a rut and at an unhealthy weight
After: two stone lighter, running half-marathons

Jacky has been a vegetarian since her teens, yet she always struggled with her weight. But it was love – and giving up smoking – that tipped the scales in the wrong direction.

'Before meeting Darren, I worked late a lot and was only cooking for myself, so most of the time it was baked potato and baked beans!

'After I met Darren, we used to go out more, have takeaways, or I used to cook and eat the same-sized portions as him. Plus, giving up smoking, I tended to replace the craving with chocolate and crisps. I didn't realise until my mum told me one Christmas that my gran had said something about how much weight I had put on.

'I went up to nearly 11 stone (154lb), and for someone who is only 5 foot 1, that is not a healthy weight to be. I tried dieting, but I couldn't stick at anything.'

But when she heard about 5:2, the idea struck a chord. 'Only dieting two days a week appealed to me. I eat healthily most of the time, but detest counting calories all week long and having to account for everything I eat and drink, so I thought I would give it a go.'

Jacky, who works as a virtual assistant, did her homework. She joined our Facebook group and read two of the 5:2 books before starting, but admits that despite the preparation, she found it daunting at first. 'The first fast was difficult. I remember watching the clock continuously. I had decided that I wouldn't eat until the main meal, so that I could take away the calorie counting as much as possible. I lived on tea and peppermint tea through the day. As time went on the fasts became easier. You realise that the hunger pangs don't last and that if you keep yourself busy, the time flies.'

And obviously, she was doing it right, because Jacky's weight fell to 8 stone 10 (114lb), though she explains, 'I do like a glass or two of wine, so have settled at just over 9 stone (126lb). Losing the weight has given me more confidence and made me more comfortable in my clothes.'

Jacky is also much more active now. 'I've started running. Before I couldn't run more than a few feet, but after losing weight and getting fitter, I have managed to run a couple of half marathons.'

It's not only Jacky who benefits from the changes. 'I live with my partner, Darren, who is not a vegetarian and won't consider going on a diet, however he does like a lot of the food that I make while on a Fast Day, so he ends up "dieting" anyway.'

Moving from Bristol to Mayenne in north-west France has been a challenge – especially as veggie food is more limited.

'I find it very difficult to go out for meals, especially on a Fast Day, as options tend to be pizza or omelettes and I have been to a restaurant and been served just vegetables! However, the options in the supermarkets are getting better and being able to get stir-fry sauces does make it easier to knock up a quick meal.'

And, of course, France has its compensations, even for a veggie. 'Luckily the French love their cheese – and so do I, but only on a non-Fast Day! I bought lots of Cheddar with me, when I arrived, and you still can't beat it for lasagne, but I also love Coulommiers, Roquefort, Emmental and Gruyère.

Fast Day routine:

One meal in the evening on most Fast Days, but occasionally a very light lunch of salad or soup, no more than 50 calories. I try to keep my calories for the main meal in the evening. I use some calories for milk in my tea and drink lots of water. If I am feeling really hungry I drink fizzy water and might even have a little bit of salad, or pickled gherkins and onions, as they just get me over that hungry 10 minutes or so.

The other 5 days:

The day after a fast, I do feel less hungry, and overall I probably eat less than I used to on those days. Bread has always been my downfall, but now I balance out meals with more veggie proteins, like pulses. It keeps me feeling fuller for longer and if I choose low-fat options, I get more for my calories. I've also become more aware of what I eat. For instance, I now eat a lot more berries and grapes in my diet, rather than bananas and dried fruit, because volume-wise they are a lot lower in calories.

The veggie life:

I have been a vegetarian for 28 years – so more than half my life – after watching a documentary on chicken farming. I do find it harder to eat protein as a vegetarian, because you have to be more mindful about your meals, and I need to soak beans overnight if they are going to form part of the meal the next day. I love experimenting with food; I'm a bit of a throw it in and see if it works kind of gal! I eat Mexican, Indian and Italian, but Indian is the easiest, as you can use lots of veggies, plus lentils are a great source of protein.

Top tips:

I would encourage anyone to try the 5:2. It's not as restrictive as other diets, there are health benefits, and it realigns your thinking by understanding that hunger pangs don't last.

Last word:

5:2 has helped me lose weight without continually feeling like I'm on a diet. I am much more comfortable in my clothes, able to exercise without difficulty, but I can still enjoy a wine or two on a non-fasting day. And the best thing is, it can be a way of life, rather than just a diet!

ARTICHOKE PÂTÉ WITH GRILLED RED CHICORY, 58 calories

This pâté is tasty, speedy and super-adaptable. Here I serve it with grilled red chicory as a tasty light lunch, but you could also serve it with very thinly sliced sourdough bread, as a pitta filling, or with salad. The beans add body and make the artichokes go further. I use a stick blender to whizz it all together in the bowl, which means minimal washing up!

Makes 330g, 4 servings of around 80g each, pâté only 51 calories
Preparation time: 8 minutes
Cooking time: 4–6 minutes (for chicory)

1 x 390g tin artichoke hearts, drained and rinsed, 72
1 lemon, 12
1 garlic clove, roughly chopped, 4
Good handful of herbs, such as basil or parsley, 5
100g cannellini beans from a tin, drained, 101
A few drops of extra-virgin olive oil, 10
2 whole red chicory, around 100g total, 27
Freshly ground sea salt and black pepper, to taste

1. Place the drained artichokes on kitchen roll to soak up any excess water.

2. Cut the end off the lemon and cut one thin slice per person, then juice the rest. Add the garlic to the beaker of a hand blender or bowl of a food processor with the lemon juice, drained artichokes and herbs. Blend well

until it forms a purée make sure the garlic is well distributed, then add
the beans and blend again to form your paste. Season well with sea salt
and pepper.

3. Heat a griddle and add a drop or two of oil. Cut the chicory in half
   lengthwise and grill for 2–3 minutes until warm, with light scorch marks.
   Serve with the pâté and lemon slices.

P. S. This is so versatile; it's delicious with 15g of olives (49
calories) added as well as the herbs, or 8g sun-dried tomatoes
(16 calories, oil removed using kitchen roll). You can also warm
it through gently before serving.

ROCKET AND RICOTTA FRITTATA MUFFINS, 79 calories per muffin

Italian frittata omelettes are quick, and make brilliant individual 'muffins'. This recipe combines dark rocket leaves with smooth ricotta cheese, plus a topping of crunchy Grana Padano. Use baking parchment or muffin cases to line muffin tins to make the finished bakes easy to transport!

Makes 6 muffins
Preparation time: 10 minutes
Cooking time: 20–25 minutes

4 eggs, 264
3 spring onions, finely chopped, 6–9
40g rocket, roughly chopped, 10
100g ricotta, 134
15g Grana Padano cheese, 58
Freshly ground sea salt and black pepper, to taste

Optional: good pinch of dried Italian herbs, 3

1. Preheat the oven to 180°C/350°F/Gas mark 4. Line the holes in a muffin tin with 1–2 small squares each of greaseproof or baking paper.

2. Mix together the eggs, onions, rocket and ricotta in a bowl, reserving 40g of the ricotta. Season, then spoon equal quantities of the mix into each of the muffin holes. Finally, place a teaspoon of the reserved ricotta into the centre of each muffin, then sprinkle the cheese over the top of each, along with the dried herbs, if using.

3. Bake for 20–25 minutes, until the tops are golden brown, then leave to cool. These are delicious eaten hot but can also be stored in the fridge for up to 3 days and microwaved for 20–30 seconds each to warm through before serving. Or you can freeze them each individually once cold then thaw before reheating and serving.

P. S. Instead of the rocket, try the same weight of baby spinach cooked and very well drained (10 calories) and 8g sun-dried tomatoes (16 calories). A great gluten-free option is the dukkah from page 249, half added to the mix and the rest sprinkled on top.

MINTY BEETROOT CAVIAR WITH RAINBOW CRUDITÉS, 113 calories

This is a spectacular and super-fast dip: deep crimson, flecked with bright green mint, flavoured with cumin and served with a rainbow plate of crudités. The garlic and yogurt are great together, but you can leave out either or both if you prefer. I always use vacuum-packed beetroot in water here so I can make this in a flash.

Makes 2 servings
Preparation time: 8 minutes

For the caviar: 58 per serving without yogurt and garlic, 67–75 with yogurt and garlic

1 x 250g pack beetroot in water, drained, 106

Handful of mint leaves, 5, reserve one for garnish

½ teaspoon ground cumin, 3

Squeeze of lemon juice, 2

Freshly ground sea salt and black pepper, to taste

Optional: 1 garlic clove, 4

Optional: 1 level tablespoon Greek or coconut yogurt, 14–29 depending on variety

To serve (crudités for 2): 46 per person

75g radishes, halved, 7

1 medium carrot, cut into batons, 34

50g sugar snap peas, halved lengthwise, 21
1 yellow pepper, deseeded and sliced into strips, 30

1. Cut the beetroot into chunks and add to a food processor with the mint leaves, cumin, garlic (if using) and a squeeze of lemon juice. Process well and add more juice if you prefer a more liquid texture. Season.

2. Spoon the dip into a serving dish and swirl through the yogurt, if using. Top with a mint leaf and serve on a platter with the prepared crudités.

P. S. Great with the falafel on page 241, or served with the lentils and labneh as part of a mezze spread. Swirl in a teaspoon of tahini (30 calories) for a nutty flavour and silkier texture.

CHESTNUT, LEEK AND MUSHROOM 'SAUSAGE' ROLLS, 144 calories

These are tasty, portable and easy to make. My neighbour, Tina, said she wishes they served these for veggies at parties instead of fake meat, soya sausage rolls. The filling is deeply savoury and the golden pastry has crunch without being heavy. Do calorie-count the pastry for these, as filo sheet sizes vary; the counts here are for a 25g sheet per mushroom roll.

Makes 4 sausage rolls (144 calories each)
Preparation time: 10 minutes
Cooking time: 25–30 minutes

2 small leeks, around 200g, chopped, 62
½ teaspoon butter or rapeseed/groundnut oil, 13/21
300g chestnut mushrooms, chopped, 60
1 teaspoon dried or chopped fresh thyme, 5
100g vacuum-packed chestnuts, roughly chopped, 106 (the rest can be frozen)
4 sheets filo pastry, around 100g (look for vegan-friendly filo), 290
1 teaspoon rapeseed/groundnut oil for brushing, 41
Freshly ground sea salt and black pepper, to taste

1. Preheat the oven to 200°C/400°F/Gas mark 6.

2. Fry the leeks in the butter or oil for 1 minute, then add the mushrooms and thyme and fry for another 4–5 minutes.

3. Pulse the chestnuts in a food processor, then add the cooked mushroom mix and pulse to form the sausage filling. Season with salt and pepper.

4. Use one pastry sheet per roll: fold the sheet in half lengthways. Place a quarter of the filling in the centre of the pastry and spread it along the length. Roll up the pastry from the long sides to create a roll. Use a pastry brush to coat the pastry with oil on both sides, then place on a baking tray and repeat to make the other rolls.

5. Once all the rolls are prepared, bake them in the oven for 20–25 minutes, checking them every few minutes towards the end of the cooking time to ensure the pastry doesn't burn. If it starts to catch, cover the rolls lightly with foil.

6. Cut the long rolls into three smaller rolls, if you like, and serve fresh from the oven, with the purple chilli kimchi-kraut on page 274, hot chilli sauce, or a salsa from page 138.

P. S. For a luxurious addition, brush the uncooked rolls with truffle oil in place of rapeseed before baking. You can also top the filling with a little crumbled goat's cheese (25g, 63–83 calories) before rolling up and baking. The rolls can be frozen: freeze after rolling but before brushing with oil. Wrap each one individually in cling film to freeze, then unwrap and cook from frozen: brush with oil and bake for 25–30 minutes or until golden brown on the outside and cooked through inside.

SUPER-SAVOURY MISO AUBERGINE, 163 calories

If you like Marmite, Vegemite or umami flavours, you'll love this. Don't be put off by the list of ingredients, the only essential one if you're new to Japanese food is the miso. Meat-eaters and aubergine-phobes will be converted by this dish.

Serves 1
Preparation time: 5 minutes
Cooking time: 25–30 minutes

1 large aubergine, around 300g, 60

For the miso marinade

2cm/5g piece fresh ginger, peeled and grated, 4
15g brown rice miso, 25
½ teaspoon honey, 10, or agave nectar, 8
10–15ml rice or white wine vinegar, 3
1 teaspoon sesame or rapeseed/groundnut, 41

For the topping

3 small spring onions, 6
½ teaspoon sesame seeds or gomasio (ground sesame condiment), 16

1. Preheat the oven to 200°C/400°F/Gas mark 6.

2. Slice the aubergine in half lengthwise, keeping the stalk intact. Cut into the flesh diagonally both ways (without slicing through the bottom) to form a cross-hatch pattern. Place in a baking dish.

3. Make the marinade by combining all the ingredients in a small bowl. Use a pastry brush or the back of a spoon to spread the marinade over the cut length of the aubergines, pushing it into the gaps. Snip the white parts of the spring onion over the top, reserving the green ends.

4. Bake in the oven for 25–30 minutes. Serve hot from the oven or at room temperature, adding the green spring onion ends as a garnish on top.

P. S. If you'd like a side dish with this, serve with the Sesame sea vegetable salad from page 270. You could also mix up more than one portion of the marinade and keep the remainder in a pot in the fridge for a couple of weeks to use on tofu, or when roasting or grilling vegetables such as courgettes, sweet potatoes or portobello mushrooms.

PACKED LUNCH PEPPER AND KALE MISO NOODLES, 247 calories

(⏺)(🥕)(🌾) if using 100% buckwheat/non-wheat noodles

Sometimes you need a super-satisfying packed lunch, and this fits the bill. Make the dressing in the lunchbox and blanch the veggies in the noodle water to cut down on time and washing-up. I promise you won't feel like you're fasting... (This also works great as a family supper dish.)

Serves 1
Preparation time: 10 minutes
Cooking time: 10 minutes (at the same time as preparing)

40g soba or buckwheat noodles, around 138 calories
10g/1 dessertspoon miso paste, 16–20
½ teaspoon sesame, olive or other nut oil, 21
20ml/2 dessertspoons rice wine vinegar, 2
1 small carrot (around 40g), cut into matchsticks, 14
30g mangetout, left whole, or sugar snap peas, cut in half, 12/10
½ red pepper, deseeded and cut into matchsticks, 15
20g baby kale leaves (or kale with the stems removed), 10
1 spring onion, 2
3g raw or salted peanuts, 17

1. Cook the noodles according to the packet instructions – usually around 10 minutes.

2. Combine the miso, oil and vinegar in the lunchbox.

3. In the last 2 minutes of cooking, add all the vegetables except the pepper, baby kale and spring onion to the noodle water to blanch. Drain the veg and noodles well and place while still warm into the lunchbox, along with the red pepper and kale. Replace the lid and give it a good shake to coat everything with the dressing.

4. Snip the spring onion onto the salad, then chop the nuts or pound in a pestle and mortar and sprinkle over. Eat warm or when cooled.

P. S. Any bite-sized veggie pieces work here: try baby sweetcorn or tiny broccoli florets in place of the carrot or peas. Just add to the simmering noodles for long enough that the vegetables are cooked al dente, or use raw.

ONION BHAJI LUNCHBOX OMELETTE, 179 calories

This is a combination of a Spanish tortilla and an onion bhaji – it produces a thick quiche-like omelette that you can slice into wedges to take to work. What's not to love? It's a little fiddly, but follow the instructions and it's lots of fun to make. As with other tortillas, it's the ultimate sandwich filler for the day after a fast, too, if you like a hearty sarnie.

Makes 4 wedges, 179 calories each
Preparation time: 5 minutes
Cooking time: 21–25 minutes (plus 15 minutes for potatoes if not parboiled)

2 small onions, thinly sliced, 76
10g butter, 72, or 2 teaspoons coconut/rapeseed/groundnut, 82
250g potatoes, parboiled with skin on and cut into thin slices lengthwise, 213
2 small red or green chillies, or 1 of each, chopped, 8
1 teaspoon garam masala, 5
1 teaspoon ground turmeric, 5
5 eggs, 330
Handful of coriander leaves, chopped, 5
Freshly ground sea salt and black pepper, to season

1. Fry the onions in a non-stick omelette pan in ½ teaspoon of butter or oil for 8–10 minutes until they're brown and crispy but not burned. Tip onto a plate lined with kitchen roll.

2. Now fry the potatoes in another ½ teaspoon of fat, with the chopped chillies and ground spices. Cook for 4–5 minutes, allowing the slices to brown slightly. Tip these onto another plate. Meanwhile, beat the eggs and add the coriander, some salt and pepper and half the onions.

3. Melt 1 teaspoon of butter or oil in the same frying pan and arrange the cooked potatoes across the pan, so they're layered and the same height. Now pour in the egg mix and tip the pan so it runs between the potato slices. Cook over a medium-high heat for 5–7 minutes, until the bottom of the omelette is brown but not burned and the egg mixture is more set. Now layer the rest of the onions on top.

4. Place a plate that's larger than the frying pan over the pan and turn the pan upside down, so the uncooked side of the tortilla ends up face down on the plate. Now slide the uncooked side back into the pan and cook for 4–5 minutes. Alternatively, if your pan is heatproof you can finish the top off under the grill. If you're going to eat this all hot, it's nice to leave the eggs slightly runnier. Otherwise let them set well.

5. Eat hot or cold with salad leaves and a little mango chutney!

P. S. Try sweet potato instead of the white: you could use paprika in place of the Indian spices, or mix in chopped oregano or thyme, for a different flavour.

MUSHROOM AND CHILLI JAM QUESADILLA, 213, with pop-art coleslaw, 52

My favourite Mexican-style snack – a melted cheese and bean sandwich. It becomes Fast Day-friendly thanks to smaller amounts of strong-flavoured ingredients. Serve with the pop-art coleslaw!

Serves 1
Preparation time: 3 minutes
Cooking time: 6 minutes

    50g chestnut mushrooms, chopped, 11
    ½ teaspoon rapeseed/groundnut oil, 21
    30g black beans, drained, from a tin or vacuum pack, 33
    1 corn or wheat tortilla, 111
    1 teaspoon chilli jam (or use chilli or tomato chutney), 19
    10g reduced-fat feta, 18
    Freshly ground sea salt and black pepper, to taste

For the pop-art coleslaw
    50g red cabbage, thinly sliced 13
    1 small carrot, around 75g, grated, 26
    1 tablespoon natural yogurt, 11–20
    ¼ teaspoon mustard or nigella seeds, 2

1. Fry the mushrooms in the oil over an intense heat so they lose all their moisture. Take the pan off the heat and add the drained black beans, and stir together. Season.

2. Spread half the tortilla with the chilli jam or chutney, add the mushroom and bean mix, crumble over the feta then fold the tortilla in half. Using the same frying pan, cook the folded quesadilla on one side over a medium-high heat until browned, around 2 minutes – it helps to press down on it with your spatula. Flip over to brown the other side and cook for another 1–2 minutes, so the cheese melts and the filling is warmed through.

3. Meanwhile, mix the red cabbage and carrot in a bowl with the yogurt and seeds. Pack into a small cup, then upend onto a plate.

4. Cut the cooked sandwich into four triangles, and serve with the coleslaw.

P. S. For a French-inspired version of this, use a milder goat's cheese with chutney or a red onion marmalade and some puy lentils or other cooked pulses.

PEACAMOLE MINT TOSTADAS WITH RED PEPPERS, 218 calories

If you love peas, you'll adore this: it tastes of the garden, with a little chilli heat, and it's so colourful, too. Tostadas are usually fried, but griddling crisps them up without needing fat.

Serves 1
Preparation time: 8 minutes
Cooking time: 10 minutes

75g frozen peas or petit pois, 45–60 calories
1 jalapeño from a jar, finely chopped, 6
1 spring onion, finely chopped, 2
Leaves from 1–2 sprigs of mint, finely chopped, 2
½ teaspoon chilli flakes, 3
1 roasted red pepper from a jar, or 2 small peppadew
    peppers, drained, 30
1 corn tortilla, 111
15g lettuce, 3
Freshly ground sea salt and black pepper, to taste
½ teaspoon toasted sesame seeds, 16, to serve

1. Prepare the filling. Cook the peas according to the packet instructions, then drain.

2. Combine the chopped jalapeño, spring onion, mint and chilli flakes with the cooked peas using a fork or a mortar from a pestle and mortar to crush lightly into a paste. Season well, and chill.

3. Remove any excess oil or water from the peppers by draining on kitchen roll, then slice into thin strips.

4. Cut the tortilla into 4–5 rounds using a pastry cutter or kitchen scissors – they don't need to be perfectly round! Cut the leftover scraps of tortilla into smaller pieces.

5. Heat a griddle and toast the rounds and pieces until browned and crispy, a couple of minutes on each side. Spread the pea paste onto the tortillas and top with pieces of red pepper. Serve alongside the lettuce, topped with the remaining peppers and 'chips'. Sprinkle over the sesame seeds to serve.

P. S. The peacamole can also be mixed with regular guacamole to help the more expensive avocado version go further! Or use in nachos on a non-Fast Day, with black beans, salsa and grated Cheddar or vegan cheese.

PUY LENTIL STUFFED RAMIRO PEPPERS, 258,
with lime pickled onions, 26 calories

I love pointy ramiro peppers, they have thinner skins than sweet peppers so they don't need pre-baking, and the twisted shapes look great on the plate. Here I keep the stuffing simple with quick-to-cook puy lentils and a creamy goat's cheese: the vegan version uses mixed seeds. Good for serving two people, or serve it hot one day for one person and keep the rest for a packed lunch/salad dish the next day. The pink pickles are deliciously piquant next to the earthy lentils and keep for 3–4 days in the fridge if you want to make extra.

Serves 2
Preparation time: 10 minutes
Cooking time: 38–40 minutes (or 17–20 if using pre-cooked lentils)

80g uncooked puy lentils, 260 (or use 175g from a pre-cooked pouch, 252 calories)
1 bay leaf, 0
2 long ramiro peppers, around 100g each, 80
½ teaspoon rapeseed or groundnut oil, 21
2 garlic cloves, chopped or crushed, 8
1 red or green chilli, deseeded and finely chopped, 4
1 teaspoon ground cumin, 5
6 cherry tomatoes, cut in half, 18–30
45g mild goat's cheese or 20g mixed seeds, 120

For the lime pickled onions, 26 per serving

1 red onion, finely sliced into rings, 38
½–1 red chilli, deseeded and finely chopped, 2–4
Juice of 1 lime, 12

1. First make the pickled onions. Place the onion in a bowl with the chopped chilli, then pour over the lime juice and set aside.

2. Rinse the lentils and place in a pan with the bay leaf and enough water to cover. Bring to the boil, then reduce to a simmer and cook for 20–25 minutes, until tender but with some bite. Drain.

3. Preheat the oven to 200°C/400°F/Gas mark 6. Cut the peppers in half lengthwise, keeping the stalk, and carefully scoop out any seeds and membranes.

4. Fry the garlic and chilli gently in the oil with the cumin for 2–3 minutes. Add the cooked puy lentils and mix everything together.

5. Divide the lentil mix between the four pepper halves: press 3 of the tomatoes, cut side up, into each of the peppers. Top with goat's cheese or seeds.

6. Bake in the oven for 15–20 minutes until the cheese has melted. Serve with the pickled onions on the side.

P. S. You can use any other cheeses, nuts or pulses with this basic recipe; try black beans with feta, or cannellini beans mixed with Italian herbs and topped with a few pine nuts.

BEANY BUNNY, AKA CURRY SANDWICH, 268 calories

I love sandwiches and I love curry, so this fun, portable lunch gets a double thumbs-up from me. Bunny chow is a South African dish that reflects the spicy packed lunches originally eaten by workers from India. It's a hollowed-out bread roll, full of a mild, slightly sweet curry. You should fill the bread only on the day you're planning to eat it, although the curry itself freezes well.

Serves 4
Preparation time: 8 minutes
Cooking time: 25 minutes

    1 teaspoon coconut or rapeseed oil, 41
    1 onion, chopped, 38
    2 garlic cloves, chopped, 8
    ½–1 green chilli, 2–4
    1 teaspoon ground cumin, 5
    1 teaspoon turmeric, 5
    1 teaspoon ground coriander, 5
    1 small potato, about 100g, diced, 80
    400g mixed vegetables: green beans, carrots, cauliflower,
        peppers, all cut into bite-sized chunks, 100–140
    ½ x 400g tin chopped tomatoes, 40
    1 x 400g tin chickpeas, drained, 312
    1 tablespoon mango or tomato chutney, 33

4 crusty rolls (when dough removed, weight for each roll is
   45g), 396
1 teaspoon coriander or nigella seeds, 5, to garnish

1. Heat the oil in a large non-stick saucepan and fry the onion, garlic, chilli, spices, and any root vegetables you are using for 5 minutes.

2. Add the remaining veggies to the pan, except those that have very short cooking times, such as green beans. Add the tinned tomatoes, chickpeas, chutney and enough water to cover the veggies. Bring to a simmer and cook for around 20 minutes, or until the potato and other root vegetables are tender.

3. Meanwhile, cut a small 'lid' off the top of each roll and carefully scoop out the dough from inside, leaving thick-enough walls to create a bread 'lunch box' (use the bread as breadcrumbs, these can be frozen).

4. Once the curry is ready, place one roll on each serving plate and spoon the curry into the centres, topping with the lids. There will be curry left over, so divide it between the plates or put it in a separate container if you are taking it to work for lunch. Top with the whole seeds.

P. S. You can use any beans for this, and you can mix and match the vegetables depending on the season or your preferences. The curry also makes a great side or main dish without the bread.

SALSAS

I love salsa, it's the perfect accompaniment to a sandwich, wrap or stuffed vegetable. Make a few portions and you can keep them in the fridge in a clean jar or plastic container for 1–2 days.

Easy salsa, makes 2 servings, 20 per serving

    3 small spring onions, chopped, 6
    1 jalapeño, chopped, 6
    2 small ripe tomatoes, chopped, 25
    1–2 tablespoons white wine vinegar, 2–4

Fruity salsa, makes 4 servings, 22–35 per serving

    200g melon, pineapple or mango, peeled and diced
        (68 calories for honeydew melon, 100 for pineapple,
        120 for mango)
    2 spring onions, chopped, 4
    1 red chilli, deseeded and finely chopped, 4
    Juice and zest of ½ lime, 8
    Handful of coriander or parsley, chopped, 5
    Freshly ground sea salt and black pepper, to taste

1. Combine the chopped fruit or veg and onions, and mix with the other ingredients in a bowl. Season to taste with sea salt and black pepper.

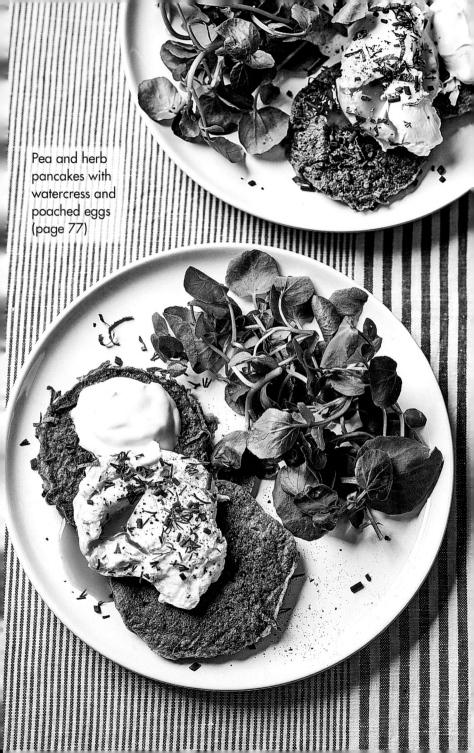

Pea and herb pancakes with watercress and poached eggs (page 77)

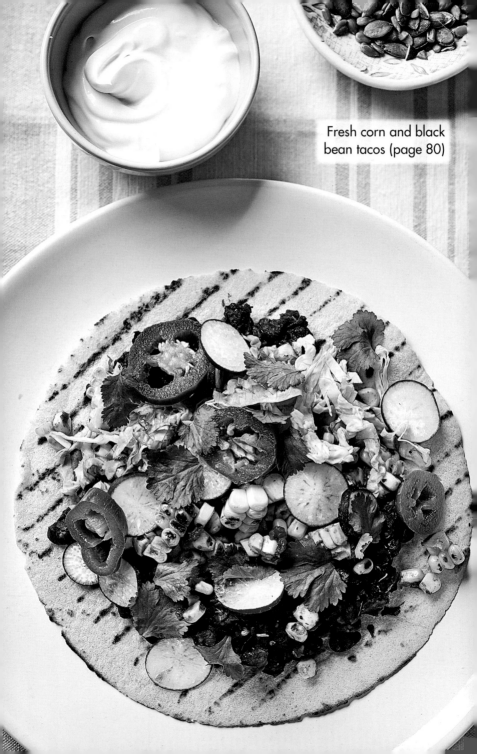

Fresh corn and black bean tacos (page 80)

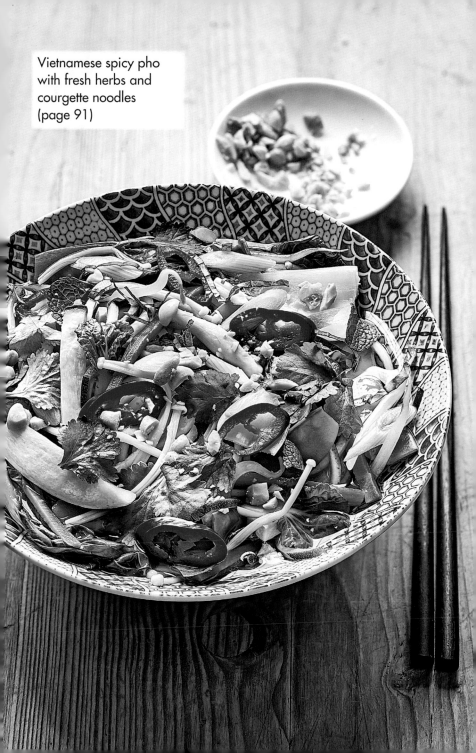

Vietnamese spicy pho
with fresh herbs and
courgette noodles
(page 91)

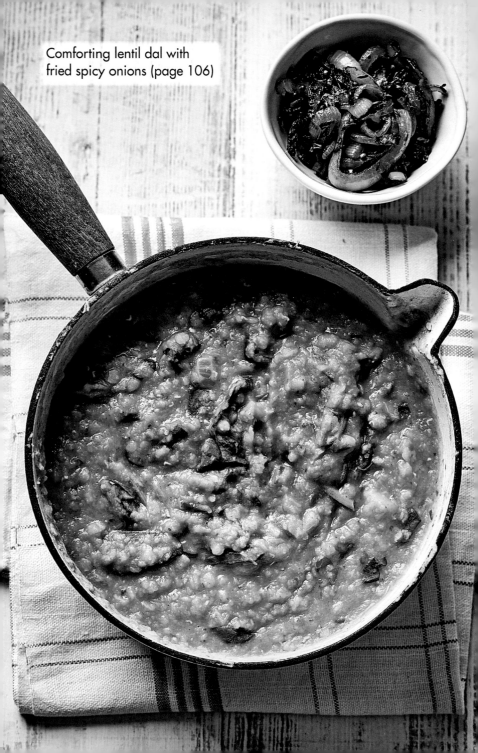

Comforting lentil dal with
fried spicy onions (page 106)

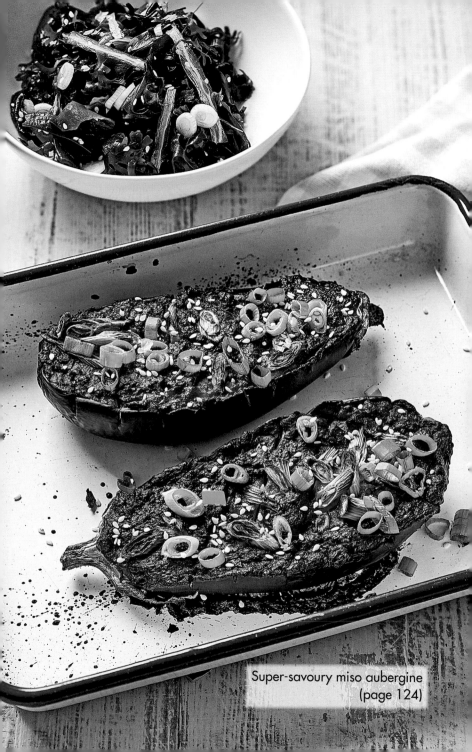

Super-savoury miso aubergine
(page 124)

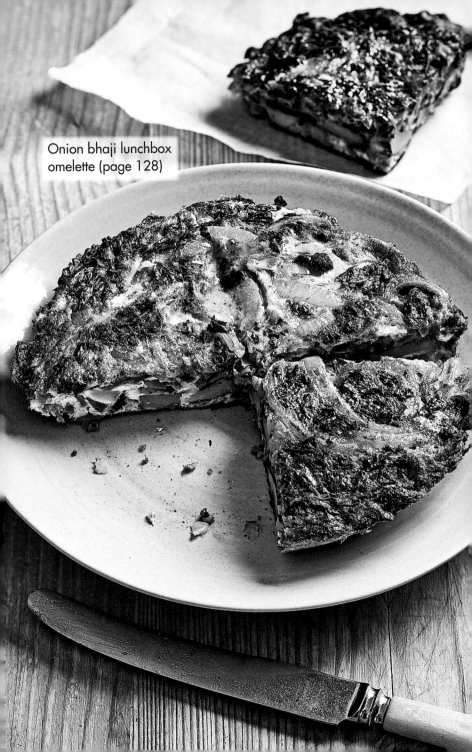

Onion bhaji lunchbox
omelette (page 128)

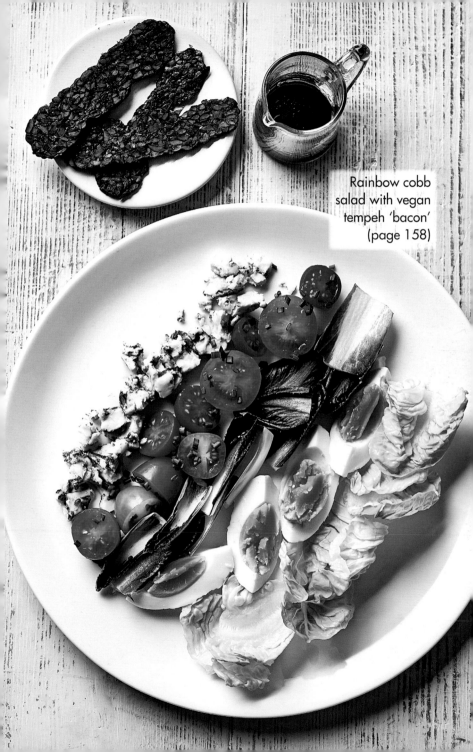

Rainbow cobb
salad with vegan
tempeh 'bacon'
(page 158)

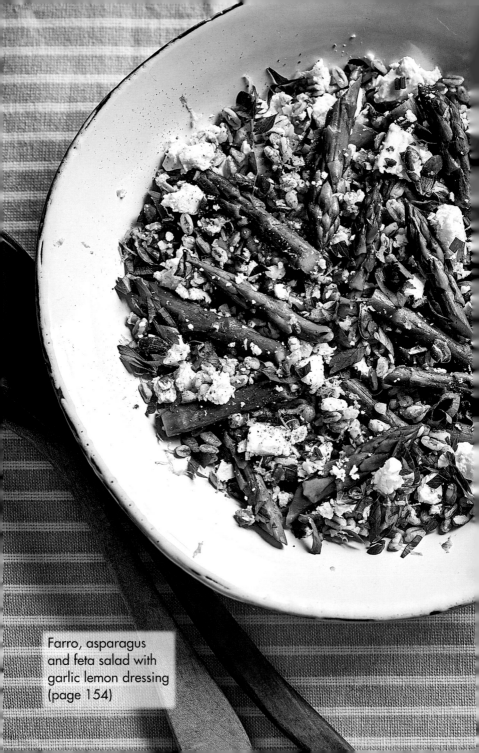

Farro, asparagus and feta salad with garlic lemon dressing (page 154)

Smoked pepper salsa, makes 4 servings, 50 per serving
This is slightly more involved, but it's worth it for its deep, smoky flavour. Dried chipotles or chipotle paste are on sale in larger supermarkets – or Amazon stock them too.

1 dried chipotle pepper, 23, or chipotle paste to taste
    (1 teaspoon is around 8 cals)
2 medium red peppers (or use 2 roast peppers from a jar, well drained), 60
4 small ripe tomatoes, finely chopped, 40
1 red onion, finely chopped, 38
½ small cucumber, 14, and ½ small stick celery, 3, finely chopped
1 garlic clove, crushed, 4
Juice of 1 lime, 12
Handful of coriander or flat leaf parsley, 5

1. Soak the chipotle in a little water to rehydrate, if using a dried pepper. Cut the fresh peppers in half, place on a baking sheet and grill until charred. Put in a bowl to cool, then remove the seeds and stalks, and peel off the blackened parts of the skin.

2. Drain the water from the chipotle and remove the stalk and seeds. Wash your hands afterwards – dried peppers are still very hot and spicy.

3. Mix all the veggies together in a bowl (add the chipotle paste now, if using paste instead of dried), add the lime juice and chopped herbs and season with black pepper.

CHAPTER FOUR

Salad

There's so much more to salad than watery iceberg lettuce. These dishes are bursting with flavour and most are also portable, so great for lunch on the go. My favourite? Tricky, but it might just be the panzanella – simple, ripe ingredients, served just right.

RECICES

CARROT AND LEMON HUMMUS SALAD JAR, ⊕⊘⊛, 140

PEACH AND TOMATO PANZANELLA, ⊕, 185

HALLOUMI SALAD WITH MELON, CUCUMBER AND MINT,
⊕⊛, 203

WARM BELUGA LENTILS WITH HOMEMADE YOGURT CHEESE,
⊕⊛, 255

FARRO, ASPARAGUS AND FETA SALAD WITH
GARLIC LEMON DRESSING, ⊕, 256

GREEN GODDESS BOWL, ⊕⊘⊛, 266

RAINBOW COBB SALAD WITH VEGAN TEMPEH 'BACON',
⊕⊘⊛, 271/336

FREEKEH PILAF WITH OLIVES, GOAT'S CHEESE & HERBS,
⊕⊘⊛, 280

BLACK RICE SALAD WITH BEETROOT, ORANGE & KEFIR,
⊕⊘⊛, 287

HEDGEROW SALAD WITH BLUE CHEESE AND BLACKBERRIES,
⊕, 361

EASY DRESSINGS

5:2 Lives

SUZANNE'S LIFE ON THE OCEAN WAVE

'I definitely feel better about my body.'

Before: tighter clothes, unhelpful food habits
After: lighter, healthier, guilt-free

Sailing to the Caribbean sounds like the idyllic life, but it came at a cost for Suzanne Wentley. 'Last January my boyfriend Brad and I left the United States for the Bahamas. Months of boat life, which included snacks, drinks and less activity, resulted suddenly in my clothes getting tight! I only have a small cubby for my clothes, and I couldn't go to the mall and buy a new size. It was time to face the music.'

An article in the *New York Times* about intermittent fasting gave her the inspiration to try 5:2. 'Something needed to happen. Living on the boat, I couldn't do programmes where you had to measure your food in little plastic boxes or eat certain "frankenfoods" as meal replacements, because I didn't have the space or even the ability to receive mail! 5:2 seemed like a simple way to take the power back, feel better about myself and just feel better in my clothes.'

Suzanne, who is 39, took the decision to begin. 'The first few Fast Days were challenging. I started to realise how I would take breaks – I work as a writer and marketing

professional online – by having a snack. I realised the amount
of alcohol I was drinking. I noticed how I'd have a sugary
dessert almost every night, because my boyfriend would.
It was a real eye-opener to understand my food habits.'

Yoga teacher Suzanne found that her practice helped her
stay on track. 'At first it didn't seem "fair" that I had to fast just
to be like everyone else. My belly rumbled so often I would
awaken at night. Still, I stuck with it. Yoga teaches you to
connect body and mind. The 5:2 diet does that as well. I just
completed my ninth month on 5:2. I do not own a scale, but
what I can tell you is that my clothes fit great now. My pants
are not falling off – though I did need an extra notch on my
belt this weekend. I still drink and eat whatever I want – just
5 days a week now instead of 7.'

More important than the weight loss is the lack of guilt:
'With 5:2, the guilt is gone. If I drink a pina colada on a non-
Fast Day, it's OK. If I eat a piece of birthday cake, it's fine.
I might not lose weight that week, even with two Fast Days,
but I'm not gaining weight either. I feel completely in control
of my weight, perhaps for the first time in my adult life.'

Fast Day routine:

Black coffee in the morning and try to last as long as possible
without any food. By 1 or 2pm I will eat half a protein bar,
or maybe an egg. Then around 3 or 4pm I will have a green
salad with red wine vinegar as dressing. This puts me at
around 140 calories. I start thinking of my options: veggie
burger, a huge bowl of miso soup with tofu and cabbage,
steamed tofu and vegetables are frequent options. It depends

what I have on the boat. Sometimes I'll just have a very small portion of whatever my boyfriend is making.

The other 5 days:

I tend to eat a smaller amount of food naturally; I drink less alcohol and snack less. I learned when I was eating out of boredom and exhaustion instead of hunger. At first, I counted calories on non-Fast Days to fully understand my relationship with food. But I eventually stopped. Now I barely think about what I am eating on non-Fast Days. I certainly still eat treats. I still have a sweet tooth sometimes. But who cares? I will be fasting twice during the week so a cookie isn't going to ruin me.

The veggie life:

I have been a lacto-ovo vegetarian since I was 15: I never liked meat. I just thought it was yucky, not something that humans are supposed to eat. I am a very creative cook and love to experiment. Besides a lot of salads, I cook curries and stir-fries, pasta and vegetable and lentil soups, tacos and bean dishes, and fun recipes like eggplant fritters. I enjoy homemade yogurt for breakfast with some fruit and a slice of homemade bread. Then lunch and dinner usually consists of a new recipe, as I love to eat new things. I enjoy trying local foods, such as tayote, and next I am going to make homemade corn tortillas for cheese and vegetable quesadillas.

Top tips:

I would suggest going online and becoming part of the online 5:2 community. I often find myself giving advice, because it was so helpful to me when I started.

Last word:

I understand now the amount of food that is appropriate for my body. I was eating too much before. That simple statement is one that most people who want to lose weight struggle to admit. The problem is figuring out what to do about it: 5:2 has helped. I feel better about myself – as simple as that. There was a time when I was looking at other women who were leaner than me, and I would compare myself harshly. Now I am able to look past their bodies and into their eyes, and smile.

CARROT AND LEMON HUMMUS SALAD JAR, 140 calories

Hummus is everywhere – and rightly so, it's delicious, versatile and packed full of good things. But the traditional recipe is quite high in calories from all the oil and sesame seeds. I played around with lots of versions before coming up with this one, using lemony ground sumac. I layer it up in a Kilner jar for the ultimate portable salad, but it's also great as a dip or sandwich filling.

Makes 1 salad jar and 3 servings of hummus
Preparation time: 15 minutes
Cooking time: 22 minutes

For the hummus (makes 3 servings), 92 per serving

½ teaspoon rapeseed/groundnut oil, 21
1 teaspoon sumac or ground cumin, 5
220g carrots (around 2 large or 3–4 medium), cut into chunks, 75
120g cooked chickpeas (½ x 400g tin, drained), 156
Juice of ½ lemon, 6
2 garlic cloves, 8
Freshly ground sea salt and black pepper, to taste

For the salad jar (per person/jar), 50 calories

50g crisp lettuce leaves, such as Little Gem, 8
½ small cucumber, around 100g, 14
½ red pepper, deseeded and sliced, 15
50g (4–6) cherry tomatoes, chopped, 10
1 small spring onion, chopped, 2
A few drops of balsamic vinegar, 1

1. Preheat the oven to 200°C/400°F/Gas mark 6.

2. Heat the oil in a small saucepan and add the sumac or cumin and three-quarters of the carrots. Fry gently for 2 minutes, then add enough water to cover the carrots and bring to a simmer: keep the water just topped up. Cook for around 20 minutes until the carrots are soft.

3. Place the cooked and remaining raw carrots in a food processor along with the chickpeas, lemon juice and garlic, plus plenty of sea salt and freshly ground pepper. Process until smooth.

4. Divide the hummus into 3 portions, using 1 for the salad jar (store the rest in a covered container in the fridge for up to 2 days).

5. Layer in a wide Kilner-style jar, alternating colours: leaves in the bottom, then a layer of hummus, then cucumber, red pepper, hummus and topped with cherry tomatoes, spring onion and a little balsamic vinegar.

P. S. Try ras al hanout spice blend in place of the sumac/cumin. The hummus is also delicious with a teaspoon of hot harissa sauce mixed into it.

PEACH AND TOMATO PANZANELLA, 185 calories

Simple but irresistible, the flavours of summer on a plate (I made it with our first tomatoes from the garden and swooned!). Tomato and peach are a classic combination, and I've added a little extra crunch with the bread to create a version of the traditional Italian panzanella salad.

Serves 1
Preparation time: 5 minutes
Cooking time: 3 minutes

1 teaspoon extra-virgin olive oil, 41
1 x 30g slice stale country/sourdough bread, 66
100g mixed ripe tomatoes, sliced or halved into bite-sized
    pieces, 20
1 ripe peach, cut into bite-sized pieces, 51
1 teaspoon white wine vinegar, 2
Small handful of basil leaves, 5
Freshly ground sea salt and black pepper, to taste

1. Heat a griddle and brush with a few drops of the oil (keep the rest for the dressing). Toast the bread on both sides, then tear into bite-sized chunks.

2. Arrange the tomatoes and peach pieces on a plate with the bread.

3. Mix together the remaining olive oil and vinegar in a bowl and drizzle over the salad, then scatter the basil leaves on top. Season well and serve at room temperature (ideally, wait for a few minutes to let the dressing soften the bread).

P. S. For a gluten-free version, substitute 10g of pistachio nuts (59 calories), lightly crushed, for the bread.

Add half a ball of 'light' mozzarella (100–109 calories) for a more substantial meal – it's not quite as creamy as the full-fat version, but it works on a Fast Day if seasoned well and accompanied by a tasty dressing.

HALLOUMI SALAD WITH MELON, CUCUMBER AND MINT, 203 calories

This is simple, sweet, salty and refreshing. Halloumi isn't low in calories, but it's a veggie winner and this version makes a little go a long way with the addition of watermelon, cucumber and mint.

Serves 1
Preparation time: 5 minutes
Cooking time: 5 minutes

⅓ pack/70g lighter halloumi cheese, 161
120g wedge watermelon, 23
½ small cucumber, around 100g, 14
Small handful of mint leaves, 5
Freshly ground black pepper, to taste

1. Slice the halloumi thinly and cut across the slices diagonally to form triangles (some will crumble, but don't worry). Cut the rind off the melon and slice into triangles. Slice the cucumber into batons.

2. Heat the griddle to hot then sear the halloumi without oil – cooking time varies according to brand, but it is usually 2–3 minutes on each side, until the cheese softens and has distinct grid marks.

3. Arrange the cheese, fruit and cucumber over a plate (make sure you get any charred bits of halloumi off the griddle, they're delicious!). Sprinkle the mint leaves over, season with pepper (the halloumi is already salty) and serve immediately.

P. S. Try basil leaves in place of the mint, or garnish with pink peppercorns for a citrusy note. If you feel like sweetening it up a little, a drizzle of 1 teaspoon of runny honey or pomegranate molasses is very good (20/13 calories).

WARM BELUGA LENTILS WITH HOMEMADE YOGURT CHEESE, 255 calories

Yes, you can make cheese at home – and impress your friends! Creamy labneh is made by straining yogurt through muslin or a clean J-cloth. The thicker the yogurt, the better it'll be – don't bother trying this with low-fat varieties. Beluga lentils are dark and very delicious, but you can use puy or brown lentils in their place.

Serves 2
Preparation time: 5 minutes plus 3+ hours for cheese to drain
Cooking time: 28–33 minutes (or 8–10 if using pre-cooked lentils)

For the labneh, 49–67 per serving

100ml thick Greek or Turkish yogurt, 95–130
¼ teaspoon fine salt
½ teaspoon sumac, paprika or ground cumin, 3

For the salad, 206–226 per serving

100g beluga, puy or brown lentils, 300–340 (or use 1 pack of pre-cooked lentils, 354)
1 bay leaf, 0
1 teaspoon extra-virgin olive oil, 41
1 red onion, sliced into rings, 38
Juice and zest of ½ lemon, 8
100g baby spinach, larger stems removed, 25
Freshly ground black pepper, to taste

1. Make the labneh up to 12 hours in advance. Mix the yogurt with salt and the spice of your choice. Place a fine sieve over a small bowl and lay two pieces of muslin (from fabric or cookware stores) or a clean J-cloth in the sieve. Spoon the flavoured yogurt into the centre, then draw up the corners and fix with string or a peg so you have a 'parcel' of yogurt. Leave it in the sieve and the whey will drip through the muslin, leaving behind cheese. In warm weather, keep this in the fridge. It'll take 3–8 hours to form the cheese. You can also weigh out the lentils now and soak in fresh cold water, to cut cooking time.

2. Rinse the lentils and place with a bay leaf in a saucepan, covered with 200ml water. Bring to the boil, then reduce to a simmer and cook for 20–25 minutes until the lentils are cooked but still have 'bite'. Top up water levels as the lentils cook so they don't burn.

3. Meanwhile, heat the olive oil in a non-stick pan. Fry the onion gently for 6–8 minutes, only stirring occasionally, so the edges brown but do not burn.

4. When the lentils are cooked, add the cooked onion, lemon juice and spinach to the pan and cook for 2–4 minutes, until the spinach wilts.

5. Tip the lentil mix into serving bowls. Open the cheese parcel and use a teaspoon to divide the cheese between the two plates in small rounds. (You can use the whey left in the bowl in savoury dishes in place of milk.) Add lemon zest and black pepper and serve.

P. S. This makes two portions; keep the lentils and the cheese separately in the fridge for use as a salad next day or reheat in a pan or microwave. Add the cheese just before serving. The labneh is the perfect blank canvas for any flavours: fresh herbs work brilliantly with it. You can also use the same technique to produce a thicker strained yogurt from normal plain yogurt.

FARRO, ASPARAGUS AND FETA SALAD WITH GARLIC LEMON DRESSING, 256 calories

Farro is emmer wheat – one of the older grains that some people find easier to digest than more modern wheats used in sliced bread (NB: emmer does still contain gluten so is not suitable for coeliacs). What I love about farro is its nutty flavour that acts as the perfect base for simple, strong flavours: in this case, fresh asparagus, creamy feta and a garlicky dressing (use half a teaspoon of French mustard if you don't fancy the raw garlic).

Serves 2
Preparation time: 5 minutes
Cooking time: 13–17 minutes

100g asparagus spears, 27
75g quick-cook farro, 271
1 bay leaf, 0
50g reduced-fat feta, 90

For the dressing, 61.5–62 per serving

Juice and zest of ½ lemon, 8
10ml extra-virgin olive oil, 82
1 garlic clove, crushed, 4
1 tablespoon pumpkin seeds, lightly crushed, 29
*Optional: top with a few torn basil leaves, chives or flat-leaf
    parsley, 1*

1. Bring a pan of 750ml water to the boil. Trim the ends off the asparagus and briefly cook for 3–4 minutes until just cooked (1–2 minutes if you are using fine asparagus). Remove from water with a slotted spoon.

2. Add the farro to the boiling water with the bay leaf and simmer for 10–12 minutes until the water is absorbed (or follow the packet instructions). Discard the bay leaf.

3. Cut the asparagus into pieces around 3cm long.

4. Combine the lemon juice and zest, oil and the garlic in a bowl.

5. When the farro is cooked, place in a serving dish, add the asparagus, stir in the dressing and season well. Crumble the feta over the top and scatter the crushed pumpkin seeds over the top.

P. S. For a vegan version, swap the asparagus for 100g long-stemmed or purple sprouting broccoli (32 calories), and use 100g of marinated tofu (from 115 calories, check packaging) in place of the cheese. Use quinoa instead of emmer for a gluten-free dish.

GREEN GODDESS BOWL, 266 calories

I don't buy into superfoods as a label – variety is my mantra, rather than singling out one ingredient – but this green bowl is packed with fashionable 'super' ingredients that also taste brilliant: avocado, kale, coconut oil and quinoa. A bowl like this is a flexible way to use up leftover veg, grains, etc., which cuts the cooking/prep time right down. Go green!

Serves 1
Preparation time: 10 minutes
Cooking time: 7–9 minutes' total (or none if using leftovers)

50g long-stemmed or purple sprouting broccoli, 16
½ teaspoon coconut oil, 21
50g kale, chopped, stalks removed, 20
½ baby/small avocado, around 50–60g flesh, 80–88
75g cooked quinoa or other grain, 90
1 tablespoon tamari or soy sauce, 9–15
½ teaspoon wasabi mustard, 3
4 pistachios, lightly crushed, 24
A few slices Japanese-style pickled ginger, 3
Optional: freshly ground sea salt and black pepper, to taste

1. Steam or boil the broccoli until very lightly cooked, 7–9 minutes. Melt the coconut oil in a pan and cook the kale for 2–3 minutes until bright green and slightly crispy. Cut the avocado flesh into cubes (if you're not planning to serve immediately, sprinkle with a little lemon juice to stop it going brown).

2. Arrange the avocado, kale, broccoli and quinoa in a bowl and pour over half the soy or tamari sauce. Serve the wasabi on the side on a spoon – beware, it's hot stuff! Sprinkle over the nuts and pickled ginger and season with more tamari/soy and sea salt and pepper, if you like.

P. S. You can include all *your* favourites in your bowl, but to get a nutritious balance, I like to include:

Protein: quinoa is a seed, not a grain, so contains protein, but you can also use nuts and seeds (sparingly) or cooked beans, such as black beans or chickpeas, or marinated or cooked tofu.

Grains/carbs: try cooked barley, farro, brown rice or cooked butternut squash/sweet potato.

Green veg: kale, spinach, broccoli and rocket all give that bitter green kick.

Sour: citrus or vinegars are great to dress your veg and grains.

Other produce: try fresh or roasted peppers, tomatoes, or fresh or dried berries.

Fat: a little fat is good for you. Avocado is a good source, as are olive and coconut oils and nut butters or tahini: but don't use too much on a Fast Day.

Flavours: garlic, ginger, chilli, fresh herbs, spices, mustard, pickled vegetables, kimchi – mix it up to match your mood and what you have in the fridge/cupboard.

Use the calorie counter on page 344 to add up the ingredients in your version and don't forget you can add more flavour with the dressings on pages 168–70!

RAINBOW COBB SALAD WITH VEGAN TEMPEH 'BACON', 271–336 calories

Veggie version with egg and blue cheese: 271
Vegan version with avocado and smoked tofu: 336

The Cobb salad is a generous main dish which was invented in Hollywood in the 1930s, and this is a veggie version, using vegan tempeh in place of bacon, but keeping the egg and blue cheese. The presentation makes it special, with all the different-coloured stripes across a plate. See more about tempeh on page 200. You can also buy ready-made vegan tempeh bacon in health food shops.

Serves 1
Preparation time: 10 minutes (plus making vegan bacon)
Cooking time: 9–11 minutes

1 egg, 66, or 40g marinated/flavoured tofu, 77
2 teaspoons red wine vinegar, 2
½ teaspoon extra-virgin olive oil, 21
1 medium flavoursome tomato or 5 cherry tomatoes, chopped into bite-sized chunks, 16–20
20g iceberg lettuce or Little Gem lettuce, chopped, 5
1 small red chicory or radicchio, leaves separated and chopped, around 40g, 9
25g Roquefort or Stilton blue cheese, crumbled, 90, or ½ small avocado, around 90g flesh, sliced, 144

1 x 25g serving homemade vegan tempeh bacon
   (see page 160), 60
Small bunch chives, 3, or 1 spring onion, chopped, 2
Freshly ground sea salt and black pepper, to taste

1. If using egg, place the egg in a small pan of cold water. Bring to the boil then simmer for 9–11 minutes, depending on how set you like your egg. When time is up, place the cooked egg in its shell into cold water, then, once it's cool enough, peel and slice.

2. While the egg is cooking, make the dressing by combining the vinegar, oil and seasoning in a bowl.

3. Arrange each ingredient in 'stripes' across the plate, contrasting the colours: such as tomatoes, green lettuce, egg/tofu, chicory, blue cheese/avocado. Add the tempeh bacon on top of the lettuce. Season, then drizzle over the dressing and snip the chives or onions over the top.

VEGAN TEMPEH BACON, 60 calories

Bacon is something a lot of veggies (including me) admit to missing, even when the craving for any other meat has disappeared. This captures the smoky, savoury element I miss, and is cruelty-free, tasty, and very quick if you have a microwave. Make 4 servings and keep the remainder in the fridge for a couple of days to put in salads and sarnies. See more about tempeh on page 200.

Serves 4, 60 per serving
Preparation time: 3 minutes
Cooking time: 5–6 minutes

100g tempeh, 190
4 teaspoons soy or tamari sauce, 12–30
4 teaspoons cider vinegar, 4
1 teaspoon agave,13, or maple syrup, 17
Sea salt, to taste
½ teaspoon olive or coconut oil, 21

1. Slice the tempeh into the thinnest slices or 'rashers' you can. If it crumbles a little, it doesn't matter.

2. Place the soy or tamari, vinegar, syrup and salt in a small microwavable plastic tub, replace the lid and shake to mix. Put the tempeh pieces inside, close and turn again to coat.

3. With the lid loosely resting on the tub (to let steam escape during

cooking), microwave the tempeh for 30–40 seconds, until the liquid has almost gone.

4. When you're ready to use, melt the oil in a non-stick pan and fry the strips of tempeh over a high temperature, turning so both sides go crispy and browned, but do not burn: it'll take 2–3 minutes on each side. Serve hot, or at room temperature.

P. S. If you don't have a microwave, let the tempeh marinate in the fridge overnight before frying up with the remaining marinade in the pan.

FREEKEH PILAF WITH COURGETTES, OLIVES AND FRESH HERBS, 280 calories

Freekeh comes from the Middle East and is made from roasted durum wheat. It has a subtle, smoky, nutty taste and chewy texture. It's high in fibre and protein, as well as lutein, which helps eye health. I made this with homegrown tomatoes, each the size of a cranberry, and it was sublime.

Serves 2
Preparation time: 5 minutes
Cooking time: 20–25 minutes

80g raw wholegrain freekeh, 300
1 small, young courgette, diced, 34
1½ teaspoons extra-virgin olive oil, 63
30g green nocellara olives, stoned and chopped, 62
3 small spring onions, chopped, 6
100g cherry tomatoes (the smaller the better), halved if bigger, 20
Small handful of herbs, such as mint, parsley, basil, 5
Juice of 1 lemon, two slices reserved, 12
10g pumpkin seeds, 58
Freshly ground sea salt and black pepper, to taste
Optional: a pinch of smoked paprika

1. Place the freekeh in a saucepan with 500ml of water and a pinch of salt. Bring the water to the boil then simmer for 20–25 minutes, until the grain is cooked but still has a little bite. You can do this in advance and refrigerate until needed.

2. Fry the courgette in a small pan in ½ teaspoon of olive oil until browned or caramelised on the edges: this takes 3–4 minutes.

3. Add the chopped veg and herbs and fried courgette to the cooked freekeh, along with the paprika, if using. Season well and place on a serving dish.

4. Mix together the remaining teaspoon of oil and the lemon juice (reserve two small lemon slices to garnish) and drizzle over the freekeh. Lightly crush the seeds and sprinkle over the pilaf. Serve warm or at room temperature.

P. S. For a veggie option, on a non-fasting day, crumble over some soft goat's cheese or dairy/non-dairy feta. You can also use other vegetables, such as broad beans, broccoli, cauliflower or roasted peppers.

BLACK RICE SALAD WITH BEETROOT, ORANGE AND KEFIR, 287 calories

Vegetarian version with dairy kefir: 287
Vegan version with coconut kefir: 280

Black rice is extraordinary – it has a deep purple-black colour, a nutty flavour and a delicious aroma and flavour. The colour also gives a clue about its nutritional value – it's packed with the same phytonutrients as blueberries, and is higher in fibre than any other type of rice. Here I combine it with nitrate-rich beetroot, antioxidant orange, plus a dressing made from kefir, which is full of probiotic bacteria, and a nutty topping. For speed, I use ready-milled flaxseed which is a tasty, nutritious option. This is a regal purple feast of a salad, and tastes wonderful. You can also use other red/wild rice mixes, but it's important to use a grain which still has a bite after cooking.

Serves 2
Preparation time: 5 minutes
Cooking time: 35–40 minutes

   100g uncooked black nerone rice, 325
   1 bay leaf
   1 small orange, around 150g, 70
   2 cardamom pods, split, 2
   75ml dairy or coconut kefir, 46, or 50ml plain yogurt loosened
      with 15ml water, 41

Good pinch, ¼ teaspoon, cayenne pepper, 1
1 x 300g pack cooked beetroot in water, drained, chopped
   into bite-sized chunks, 106
A few parsley leaves, roughly chopped
Milled flaxseed/nut mix, 5g, 28

1. Rinse the rice then place in a pan with 500ml water and bring to the boil. Simmer with the bay leaf for 35–40 minutes, skimming off any foam. Drain, remove the bay leaf, and allow to cool.

2. Zest the orange and place in a small dish or jug, then peel and cut the flesh into small chunks over another bowl to catch any juice.

3. Add the cardamom pods to the orange zest with the kefir. Add the cayenne a little at a time, until it reaches the heat you like – cayenne is powerful stuff!

4. When ready to serve, mix the beetroot and rice together and arrange in a serving dish. Scatter the orange pieces on top, followed by the herbs and the ground seeds or crushed nuts. Serve the dressing on the side, to be added as you eat.

P. S. If you want to cook your own beetroot, leave it unpeeled and only remove the bigger leaves, trimming 2–3cm above the root. Simmer for 30–40 minutes (longer if the beetroots are very big) and peel while warm – do it quickly or wear gloves as it can stain your hands. Look for unusual beet varieties, like golden or candy cane. Crushed pistachios or walnuts would also taste gorgeous instead of the ground flaxseed mix.

HEDGEROW SALAD WITH BLUE CHEESE AND BLACKBERRIES, 361 calories

Autumn in a bowl: nutty barley, juicy blackberries, buttery pear, a scattering of crunchy cobnuts (available from August to October in the UK) or hazelnuts, tangy Stilton or goat's cheese all topped off with a cider vinegar honey dressing. You can cook the barley in advance or use a different, faster-cooking grain such as buckwheat or farro (see page 155).

Serves 1
Preparation time: 5 minutes
Cooking time: 35–50 minutes for the barley

   30g pearl barley or other grain, 106
   50g blackberries, 20
   40g lamb's lettuce or baby spinach leaves, 6–9
   1 small firm pear, chopped into chunks, 50
   10g shelled fresh cobnuts in season or hazelnuts, lightly
       crushed, 63
   15g crumbled Stilton, 63, or 20g soft goat's cheese, 54
   Freshly ground sea salt and black pepper, to taste

For the dressing

   1 tablespoon cider vinegar, 2
   ½ teaspoon honey, 10
   1 teaspoon olive or rapeseed oil, 41
   Pinch of sea salt

1. Cook the pearl barley according to the packet instructions, rinse and drain well, then leave to cool a little.

2. Wash the blackberries and salad leaves carefully.

3. Make the dressing by combining the ingredients.

4. Mix the barley with the lettuce or spinach and pear, and stir in half the dressing. Season well. Top with the blackberries, nuts and crumbled cheese, drizzle over the remaining dressing and serve warm or at room temperature.

P. S. This isn't just for the autumn: vary the berries and salad leaves to suit the seasons and what's in your fridge, but keep the proportions similar: for example, use raspberries, apple, almonds, freekeh (see page 161) and mature Cheddar.

EASY DRESSINGS

If I'm in a hurry on a Fast Day, I simply drizzle a little balsamic or cider vinegar on leaves, or lemon juice and maybe ½ teaspoon of extra-virgin olive oil over vegetables. But making dressings is quick and easy, and you can make them in advance and keep them in the fridge so they're ready when you need them.

Even though these dressings are generally lower in calories than those made with oil alone, they are still quite high in calories, so measure them out carefully and be sparing on Fast Days.

P. S. Dips like the Carrot and lemon hummus (page 146) or Minty beetroot caviar (page 120) can work as dressings too, especially in sandwiches or wraps.

For all the recipes below, simply put the ingredients in a clean jam jar, put the lid back on and give them a good shake. You can then keep the jar in the fridge and shake again before using. Alternatively, place the ingredients in a small bowl and whisk thoroughly until combined and smooth.

Season each with salt and pepper to taste (though bear in mind that dressings containing soy sauce will already taste quite salty).

Creamy golden dressing

A great way to get some nutrient-rich turmeric into your diet. If you don't like the flavour of turmeric, use finely chopped fresh herbs, mustard powder or just sea salt and ground pepper.

Makes: 100ml, 58
Calories per level teaspoon: 3

4 tablespoons fat-free Greek yogurt, 32
2 tablespoons cider or white wine vinegar, 4
1 teaspoon clear honey, 20, or agave nectar, 17
½ teaspoon ground turmeric (or 1 teaspoon chopped fresh herbs), 2

Sweet and sour balsamic dressing

Makes: 150ml, 223–390
Calories per teaspoon: 7–13 (NB: balsamic vinegar varies so check your label)

4 level tablespoons balsamic vinegar, 60–180
1 tablespoon light soy sauce, 9–15
1 teaspoon Dijon mustard, 5
1 tablespoon clear honey, 60
3 tablespoons fat-free Greek yogurt, 48
1–2 teaspoons extra-virgin olive oil, 41–82

Piquant Italian dressing

Makes: approx. 50ml, 275
Calories per teaspoon: 28

2 tablespoons extra-virgin olive oil, 246
1 tablespoon red wine vinegar, 3
1 teaspoon clear honey, 20, or agave syrup, 17
1 garlic clove, crushed, 4
generous pinch of chilli flakes, 1
a few finely chopped basil leaves, 1

Nutty Asian dressing

Deeply savoury and smoky. Use this sparingly, as it's high in calories. It works well on steamed vegetables, too.

Makes: 100ml, 316–358
Calories per teaspoon: 16–18

2 tablespoons sesame oil (or 1 sesame and 1 groundnut oil),
    246
4 tablespoons soy sauce, 30–72
1 garlic clove, 4
1cm piece fresh ginger, peeled and finely grated, 3
1 teaspoon toasted sesame seeds, 32
A few finely chopped coriander and basil leaves
    (Thai or normal), 1

CHAPTER FIVE

Spice

Spices, chillies, fresh herbs: this might be my favourite chapter! Try the perfect pepper stir-fry, a tangy jungle curry from Thailand, a soul-nourishing bean stew from Louisiana, and possibly the best tikka masala you'll ever have. And feel extra good knowing that many spices are the best source of compounds that can boost your immunity, fight cancer and reduce inflammation. Another fab reason to spice up your life on a Fast Day!

RECIPES

HOT AUBERGINE AND PEPPER PERFECT STIR-FRY, ⓘ ✐ ⓦ, 155

KOREAN GRILLED CAULI WITH SWEET CHILLI SAUCE,
ⓘ ✐ ⓦ, 165

SMOKY SOUL FOOD GUMBO WITH VEGAN SAUSAGE, ⓘ ✐, 200

SENEGALESE SPICY SQUASH AND PEANUT STEW, ⓘ ✐ ⓦ, 220

THAI JUNGLE CURRY WITH BABY CORN AND TOFU, ⓘ ✐ ⓦ, 238

GADO GADO INDONESIAN EGG SALAD WITH
HOT PEANUT SAUCE, ⓘ ⓦ, 252

JERK TOFU STEAKS, ⓘ ✐ ⓦ, 276, WITH COCONUT SPINACH, 35

CHICKPEA AND POMEGRANATE CHAAT STREET FOOD SALAD
WITH FRESH, FAST INDIAN HERB CHUTNEY, ⓘ ✐ ⓦ, 286

PANEER TIKKA MASALA/TOFU TIKKA MASALA, ⓘ ✐ ⓦ, 301/245

JAVANESE TEMPEH KEBABS WITH SWEET SOY MARINADE,
ⓘ ✐ ⓦ, 323

CAULIFLOWER RICE, ⓘ ✐ ⓦ, 25

5:2 Lives

LIZ'S DIAGNOSIS AND VISION
OF A 5:2 VEGAN FUTURE

'I know in my heart this is the right way to live.'

Before: 6 stone 4lb (40kg) overweight, feeling like a bloated blimp

After: slimmer, better mental health, planning for a future after cancer

It's been a rollercoaster couple of years for Liz Wakeford – she's lost 6 stone 4lb (40kg), had treatment for facial cancer, and decided to go vegan. But despite the ups and downs, she's feeling confident about the future. And 5:2 has played a big part...

When Liz first decided to try 5:2 early in 2014, she felt at a very low ebb. 'I weighed 18 stone 12lb (120kg). I was unhealthy, tired and lacked energy. I could never lose weight no matter what I did or tried, I would lose some and gain more. I had given up. I felt like a bloated blimp and very unattractive.'

But then her sister showed her a book about fasting that she'd been given by a doctor she worked with, 'and we thought, why not? Nothing else has worked. Both our husbands found this very humorous – "another diet", " here we go again" – but we still forged ahead. I felt the science behind it might just work.'

Her first Fast Day went OK except for one thing. 'I was so cold, I got the Fast Day chills. But I felt determined to keep going and give it a proper go.'

Liz, who lives in Brisbane, Australia, saw rapid results – her photos in our 5:2 group attracted many thumbs-ups – and showed on the scales and in what she wore. 'I have gone from 18 stone 12lb (120kg) to 12 stone 8lb (80kg), and from a size 22 to a size 14.'

The health improvements were life-changing, too – her high blood pressure disappeared and the bipolar disorder which affected her mood and mental health improved, with no seasonal affective disorder. Her husband Raymond also embarked on a fasting regime and lost 5 stone 7lb (35kg).

But then in January 2016, she was diagnosed with cancer on her face and had to embark on a difficult and painful course of treatment. Yet, she says, 'I feel good. I have a lot more energy and I have been able to get through the bout of cancer a lot easier than I think I would have done before.'

The illness, and an increased interest in nutrition, has prompted the two sisters to take another big step. After watching the documentary film, Forks Over Knives, they've adopted a mainly vegan diet, and Liz often makes fresh juices as meals on her Fast Days. It's another sign of how flexible 5:2 can be.

Fast Day routine:

I found Fast Days very easy from the beginning because I planned what I was eating and chose whole foods that were natural. I decided as I was doing 5:2 I would remove everything man-made as well. I love the Fast Days; so simple and easy. I mainly have vegetable and fruit juices now, at 10am, 2pm and 6pm. I feel they've helped kick-start my body after having cancer. I love juicing – I just hate washing the juicer!

The other 5 days:

I don't count calories on non-Fast Days and live on a mainly vegan diet. When I go out sometimes I may have small amounts of dairy, such as cheese and sour cream, as it's very hard to find vegan places close to home. I eat two meals: brunch and dinner, but nibble on fruit, nuts and seeds during the day. We love vegan lasagne, vegan nachos, and I make all my own vegan butters, mayo and sour creams. I make vegetable soups and lentil and chickpea burgers, and a lot of vegan Indian dishes which I serve with brown rice.

The veggie life:

5:2 made me realise the quality of my food was more important than anything else. You could effectively eat more on a Fast Day by eating healthy choices, rather than having processed man-made foods that are high in sugar, chemicals and bad fats.

The cancer diagnosis made me look into diet and nutrition, and I stumbled across some documentaries on plant-based eating. I decided that it made sense that in order to give my body the best chance of never getting cancer again, I should go vegan. I don't feel blocked up or lethargic for hours like I did after eating meat. The only thing I find hard is eating out and people's attitudes towards veganism; it's like you have grown an extra head. My hubby has joined me after watching documentaries with me, but my adult children just don't understand why we would give up meat. For me, the best thing is that I know my body feels better and lighter.

Top tips:

Remember that if you mess up there is always tomorrow. That's the best thing: one bad day can be corrected the very next day. And in general, look at what you eat and make healthier choices every day.

Last word:

So many things are better. I now box and do more general exercise. I get on my hubby's motorbike and go for rides, as I'm not afraid about being so big on it that I'll look silly. I know in my heart this is the right way to live.

HOT AUBERGINE AND PEPPER PERFECT STIR-FRY, 155 calories

So, I'm embarrassed to say that vegetable stir-fry, surely one of the simplest dishes there is, defeated me for years. But with a little research, I discovered where I was going wrong, so I'm letting you in on the tricks that I learned! This simple dish is cooked in a way you may not expect:

– the vegetables are cooked first;
– the aromatics – garlic, ginger, chilli – are cooked in a cornflour 'slurry' (much nicer than it sounds!) to create a thicker sauce;
– a little sesame oil is added at the point of serving, to intensify the flavour.

Try it out and let me know what you think. I hope you'll be very pleasantly surprised.

Serves 1
Preparation time: 8 minutes
Cooking time: 8–9 minutes

2 tablespoons water
1 tablespoon white wine vinegar, 2
1 tablespoon soy or tamari sauce, 9–18
¼ teaspoon cornflour, 10
Pinch of brown sugar, 3
1 teaspoon sesame oil, 41

1 small aubergine (230g or so), cut in half lengthwise then into
    long thin strips, 46
1 red pepper, deseeded and cut into strips, 30
2 spring onions, sliced on the diagonal, 4
1cm piece fresh ginger, peeled and grated, 2
1 garlic clove, finely chopped, 4
½ long red chilli, thinly sliced into rings, 4
A few leaves of coriander and a few sesame seeds

1. Mix together the water, vinegar, soy or tamari and cornflour in a small
   cup or dish and add a pinch of brown sugar.

2. Heat the wok, and when it's very hot, add half the sesame oil. Tip in the
   aubergine and pepper and cook for 4–6 minutes over a high heat, until
   the vegetables are softer and the edges browned. Tip them out onto a
   plate.

3. Take the wok off the heat and pour in the vinegar, soy and cornflour
   mix, followed by the spring onions, ginger, garlic and chilli. Let the sauce
   thicken for a minute or so. Now tip the vegetables back into the pan,
   return to a low heat and stir the vegetables into the sauce.

4. The stir-fry is ready. Once it's in the serving dish, pour over the other
   ½ teaspoon of sesame oil, add the coriander and sesame seeds (be
   very sparing as all seeds are nutritious but high in calories) and eat
   immediately.

P. S. Use this technique with all your stir-fries. In this dish,
baby corn makes a lovely alternative to the peppers. Serve with
cauliflower rice, page 202.

KOREAN GRILLED CAULI WITH SWEET CHILLI SAUCE, 165 calories

A Japanese yakitori grill restaurant might not seem the ideal place for a veggie, but one of my favourite places in Brighton is Bincho Yakitori, where vegetables taste amazing. This is my homage to their Korean deep-fried cauli dish: there's no deep-frying involved, but it produces the same caramelised veg with a sticky, sweet-sour sauce. I use gochugaru flakes, available from Asian grocers – and Amazon – but you can use normal chilli flakes: adjust the heat level to suit your taste.

Serves 1
Preparation time: 5 minutes
Cooking time: 9–10 minutes

- 250g cauliflower florets (around ½ large cauliflower, or a whole small one), 63
- 1 teaspoon sesame oil, 41
- Sesame seeds (white or a mix of white and black), ½ teaspoon, 16

For the Korean sauce, 40 calories

- 2 tablespoons rice vinegar, 6–10
- 1 teaspoon honey, 20, or brown sugar, 15
- ¼–1 teaspoon gochugaru or chilli flakes, 3–5
- 1 teaspoon soy or tamari sauce, 5
- 2 teaspoons tomato purée, 7–14
- 1 garlic clove, chopped, 4

1. Cook the cauliflower in boiling water until just tender, but still quite firm: this will take 3–4 minutes. When the cauli is cooked, drain in a colander and rinse under cold running water.

2. Heat a griddle and use a pastry brush to coat the florets sparingly with some of the sesame oil. Place the cauli florets on the grill pan and let them caramelise around the edges, turning them as they cook: it'll take around 5 minutes.

3. Meanwhile, place the sauce ingredients in a small saucepan, add 2 tablespoons of water and bring to a simmer. The sauce will become more concentrated and sticky as it cooks; add more water if it thickens too much, you want it to be a pouring consistency.

4. Arrange the cauliflower on a plate, pour over the hot sauce, sprinkle with the sesame seeds and eat straight away.

P. S. This is a main-course portion; serve with the Sesame sea vegetable salad from page 270 or a salad of dark, fresh leaves like rocket. I recommend making more than one portion of the sauce – it's great with so many vegetables, and also with tofu. Store in a jar in the fridge for up to a week, adding a little more water and stirring well, before heating up. The grilled cauli is also great in salads.

SMOKY SOUL FOOD GUMBO WITH VEGAN SAUSAGE, 200–231 calories

Gumbo is a spicy, Southern, slow-cooked dish using okra – green, finger-shaped veggies you might have tried in Indian dishes. So much of the flavour comes from the roux, a simple mix of flour and fat that turns the colour of dark chocolate as it cooks. Dial the cayenne up or down depending on how hot you like your food – or use a Cajun spice blend. Vegan sausages are a fab finishing touch – I used spicy chorizo-style ones made from seitan. Delicious!

Serves 4
Preparation time: 10 minutes
Cooking time: 20–25 minutes

For the roux, 86 –89.5 per serving

1 tablespoon/15g butter or rapeseed/groundnut oil, 108–123
2 level tablespoons wholewheat flour, 93
1 onion, chopped, 38
1 green pepper, deseeded and chopped, 30
1 yellow pepper, deseeded and chopped, 30
1 celery stick, chopped, 6
1 medium carrot, 100g, 31
2 garlic cloves, finely chopped, 8

For the spices, 2.75–4.3 per serving

½ –1 teaspoon cayenne or smoked paprika, 3–5

1 teaspoon dried thyme, 5
½ teaspoon allspice, 3 OR 1 teaspoon Cajun spice mix, 5

150g fresh or thawed frozen okra, stalks removed and
    chopped into rounds, 49
1 x 400g tin black-eyed beans, drained, 256
2 spicy veggie/vegan sausages, 140–250
Freshly ground sea salt and black pepper, to taste

1. Using a large, heavy-based, non-stick saucepan or casserole dish, melt the
   butter or oil with the flour and let the flour cook until it smells 'toasted'
   and changes colour to dark chocolate-brown. Watch it carefully, you don't
   want it to burn. It'll take around 10 minutes.

2. Add all the fresh vegetables except the okra to the roux, along with the
   garlic, cayenne or paprika, thyme and allspice or Cajun seasoning. Sauté
   for 3–4 minutes, then add the okra and sauté for another 2 minutes.

3. Add the black-eyed beans, plus 100ml of water. Bring to the boil,
   then reduce the heat to a simmer for 5–8 minutes until the sauce has
   thickened and the vegetables are soft. You can add a little more water if
   you prefer more sauce.

4. Meanwhile, grill or dry-fry the veggie sausages according to the packet
   instructions and then cut into pieces.

5. Season the gumbo to taste – you can add a little more cayenne if you
   like – and serve each portion topped with the sausage pieces.

P. S. Add greens such as 100g washed young spinach or kale
leaves (25–40 calories) to the dish at the end of the cooking
time and heat through until wilted.

SENEGALESE SPICY SQUASH AND PEANUT STEW, 220 calories

This is a West African dish I'd read about but never tried, and wow, was it worth making. Warming orange veggies, a cayenne pepper kick, comforting lentils and a very generous addition of peanut butter – it is delicious. You can eat it as a stew or add a little extra stock to make a fabulous soup.

Serves 4
Preparation time: 10 minutes
Cooking time: 28–30 minutes

1 teaspoon coconut or rapeseed/groundnut oil, 41

1 onion, chopped, 38

2 garlic cloves, chopped, 8

200g carrots, cut into small chunks, 68

2cm piece of fresh ginger, peeled and grated, 4

1 teaspoon curry powder or garam masala, 5

Cayenne pepper or chilli powder, 5

200g butternut squash, cut into small chunks, 80

100g red lentils, 330

500ml vegetable stock, homemade (see page 108) or made
     with 1 teaspoon vegetable bouillon powder, 12

2 tablespoons tomato purée, 10–28

½ x 400g tin chopped tomatoes, 40

40g whole nut peanut butter, 238

Optional: 100g baby spinach, larger leaves chopped, 25

1. Heat the oil in a large non-stick saucepan and fry the onion for 5 minutes with the garlic, carrots, ginger, curry powder or garam masala, and cayenne or chilli powder. Add the squash, lentils, stock, tomato purée and tinned tomatoes. Bring to the boil, simmer for around 20 minutes, stirring occasionally, until the carrots are soft and the water has been absorbed by the lentils – add a little more water if needed.

2. Stir in the peanut butter, add the spinach, if using, and warm through until the peanut butter is well mixed and the spinach is wilted. If you are planning to freeze this, do so before adding the spinach and add when reheating.

P. S. To make this into a soup, add another 500ml of water or stock after adding the peanut butter (and spinach, if using). Blend with a stick blender to the texture you prefer: I like mine smooth and silky.

THAI JUNGLE CURRY WITH BABY CORN AND TOFU, 238 calories

Some like it hot – and if that includes you, jungle curry is the one to go for. For a Fast Day, it helps that it's one of the few Thai curries that doesn't use rich coconut milk, and by making your own paste, you can leave out veggie no-nos like shrimps or fish sauce, which you'll find in many shop-bought varieties. This recipe serves 1 but the paste will make up to 3 curries.

Serves 1, 221
Preparation time: 15 minutes
Cooking time: 8–10 minutes

100g plain tofu, cut into 1cm pieces, 115
1 teaspoon coconut or rapeseed/groundnut oil, 41
100g baby corn, sliced in half lengthwise if large, 28
60g green beans, mangetout or sugar snap peas, trimmed, 20
2 teaspoons soy or tamari sauce, 6–20
¼ teaspoon palm sugar or brown sugar, 5
½ lime, to serve, 6

For jungle paste (makes 2–3 servings, 17 per serving)

2–4 small red chillies (e.g. bird's eye), depending on how hot you want your paste, deseeded, 8–16
4 garlic cloves, 16
1 lemongrass stalk, white part finely chopped, 3

3 shallots or ½ onion/red onion, chopped, 19
2cm piece fresh ginger, peeled and grated, 4
3–4 kaffir lime leaves (fine to leave out if you don't have any), 2

1. Process all the paste ingredients with a stick blender, in the small bowl of a food processor, or pound in a pestle and mortar to form a paste.

2. Set the tofu on kitchen roll to absorb as much of its water as you can.

3. Heat half the oil on a high heat in a small frying pan or wok, and fry the tofu for 3–4 minutes, turning to ensure all sides are browned. Tip out onto a plate, then add the other half of the oil to the same pan and stir-fry the corn and green vegetables for 1 minute.

4. Turn down the heat and add 2–3 tablespoons of the paste, plus the soy/ tamari, sugar and 100ml of water. Bring the mixture to a simmer and cook until the sauce thickens and the vegetables are just tender, 3–4 minutes.

5. Return the tofu cubes to the pan to warm through, then serve the curry in a shallow bowl with half a lime, to squeeze at the table.

P. S. Store the paste in a small screwtop jar in the fridge for up to 7 days (it can keep a lot longer but that's to be on the safe side).

You can add any green or root vegetables you like to this, just adjust the simmering time to ensure they're cooked but still crunchy. Serve with cauliflower rice, page 202.

GADO GADO INDONESIAN EGG SALAD WITH HOT PEANUT SAUCE, 252 calories

Gado gado is an Indonesian dish; it means 'mix-mix' and is basically a beautiful fresh main-course salad with eggs and a spicy satay-like peanut sauce. This version cheats by using ready-made peanut butter, and leaving out palm sugar and galangal, but I won't tell if you don't… It makes a great sharing dish for a summer's day. The sauce also works wonderfully on cooked veggies so consider making extra.

Serves 3
Preparation time: 20 minutes
Cooking time: 15 minutes

3 eggs, 198
150g green beans, trimmed, 41
150g pak choi, 26
100g tinned or very fresh beansprouts, 30 (see important safety warning below)
1 Little Gem lettuce, leaves separated, 15
10 cherry tomatoes, halved, 30–50
½ small cucumber, sliced into rounds, 14

For 3 servings of the sauce, 134 per serving

2 garlic cloves, finely chopped, 8
1–2 red chillies, finely chopped, 4–8
2cm piece fresh ginger, peeled and grated 4

½ teaspoon coconut oil, 21
2 tablespoons whole nut peanut butter, 179
100ml coconut milk, 178
1 tablespoon soy or tamari sauce, 9–30
100ml water
Optional: 10g peanuts, crushed, 56, to garnish

1. Boil the eggs for around 11 minutes. Allow to cool, then peel off the shells and cut the eggs in half.

2. Blanch the green vegetables: cook the green beans for 3 minutes in boiling water, then remove with a slotted spoon and use same water to blanch the pak choi for 1 minute, then the beansprouts for 1 minute.

3. To make the sauce, fry the garlic, chillies and ginger gently in the coconut oil in a small saucepan. Then add the peanut butter, coconut milk and soy or tamari sauce. Heat, stirring until well mixed. Add the water and stir until the sauce thickens.

4. Arrange the lettuce on the base of the serving dish, then pile in the blanched veg, followed by the salad veg and finally the eggs. Pour the sauce over, and sprinkle with the crushed peanuts, if using.

Important: Handle fresh beansprouts carefully because, surprisingly, they are a very common cause of food poisoning. Rinse well and discard any sprouts that are smelly, brown or even slightly musty. If you are immune-compromised or serving this to children, the elderly or pregnant women, stir-fry the sprouts in coconut oil for at least 4 minutes before serving, or use shredded lettuce instead. Tinned beansprouts can be safer and taste pretty good.

P. S. Replace the eggs with fried tofu for a vegan version (50g of tofu is 58–60 calories, check the label). Other additions that Indonesians like include boiled salad potatoes, and those *very* addictive pre-fried onions you can buy in packets (probably not for a Fast Day…).

JERK TOFU STEAKS, 276, WITH COCONUT SPINACH, 35 calories

There's a great Jamaican barbecue down the road from me, and the smell of jerk seasoning always makes my mouth water. Here, I've applied it as a marinade to tofu – the plain variety is fine – which has been pressed until it's dense and delicious.

The list of ingredients for this dish may seem daunting, so if you prefer you can buy ready-made jerk seasoning in supermarkets and add to the tomato purée and sugar: you might then feel inspired to make your own seasoning! Store any leftover marinade in a jar in the fridge for a week.

Serves 2
Preparation time: 15 minutes + pressing and marinating tofu
    (ideally overnight)
Cooking time: 10 minutes

    300g tofu, 345
    1 teaspoon coconut or rapeseed/groundnut oil, 41
    240g tomatoes, roughly chopped, 48, or 1 tin chopped
        tomatoes, 80
    1 red pepper, deseeded and roughly chopped, 30

For the DIY jerk marinade, 44–66 per serving

    3 garlic cloves, 12
    2 teaspoons allspice, 10
    Zest and juice of 1 lime, 15

1 jalapeño or Scotch bonnet if you love hot chilli, 4–6

½ teaspoon ground cinnamon, 3

2 small spring onions, 4

1 teaspoon dried thyme, 5

1 tablespoon soy or tamari sauce, 9–30

1 tablespoon tomato purée, 10–23

1 teaspoon sugar or honey, 15–20

Optional: a little grated nutmeg

1. Remove the tofu from the packaging and slice into thin rectangular 'steaks'. 'Press' the tofu: Line a plate with kitchen roll, place the tofu on top, then another sheet of roll, followed by a second plate and something heavy, such as bottles or jars. Refrigerate or keep in a cool place overnight or for a few hours – this will improve the tofu's texture.

2. Make the jerk seasoning by processing all ingredients in the small bowl of a food processor, or using a stick blender (use a deep beaker so you don't get chilli in your eye, because it's quite a dry mix). Smear the jerk seasoning thickly over both sides of each steak and let it marinate as long as you can.

3. Melt the oil on a griddle. Add the veggies to half the grill, and the tofu to the other half. Use your spatula to help break up the tomatoes to form a sauce with the peppers. Turn the tofu after 4–5 minutes, when there are stripes on one side, then cook for another 4–5 minutes.

4. Place the tomato sauce on a plate and top with the steaks, scraping any cooked marinade on top. Serve with the coconut spinach below or, on a non-Fast Day, coconut rice.

COCONUT SPINACH, 35 calories per serving

Serves 2
Cooking time: 3–4 minutes

> 150g frozen spinach, 45
> 2 teaspoons coconut cream, 24
> Grated nutmeg
> Freshly ground sea salt and black pepper, to taste

1. Cook the spinach according to the packet instructions. Season, then spoon onto a plate, stir through the coconut cream and grate a little nutmeg on top.

P. S. The jerk marinade is great on other veggie slices, try courgette or aubergine rounds. Or on a non-Fast Day, try it with halloumi cheese!

CHICKPEA AND POMEGRANATE CHAAT STREET FOOD SALAD WITH FRESH, FAST INDIAN HERB CHUTNEY, 286–296 calories

The 'street diner' held every Friday right near me in Brighton is a brilliant source of ideas and great food. I love the Honeycomb Cake brownies on a non-fasting day, but there was no way to make those Fast-Day friendly! Instead, I adapted a salad from the Ahimsa veggie stall. I've cut out the puffed rice and added more veg, nuts and a kefir dressing – made from fermented milk with lots of friendly bacteria. You can use coconut yogurt or coconut kefir to make the dish vegan. Use fresh herbs or the mint chutney over the page for an even zingier salad.

Serves 2
Preparation time: 5 minutes

    1 x 400g tin cooked chickpeas, drained and rinsed, 312
    ½ red onion, finely chopped, 38
    100g cooked new potatoes, diced, 80
    1 red or yellow pepper, deseeded and finely chopped, 30
    3–4 radishes, sliced thinly, 3
    9 almonds or 10 pistachios, lightly crushed 60
    2 tablespoons pomegranate seeds, 24
    2 tablespoons kefir, or natural/coconut yogurt thinned with a
        little milk, 17
    ½ teaspoon chilli flakes or chilli powder (or more/less to taste), 3

Chopped handful of fresh coriander and mint or mint chutney
    (see age 194), 5
Freshly ground sea salt and black pepper, to taste

1. Simply combine all the ingredients in a bowl. Season well. If you're
   taking this for lunch, keep the sauce/herbs and kefir separate and add
   just before serving.

FRESH, FAST INDIAN HERB CHUTNEY,
5–10 calories per serving

This is a good way to use fresh herbs and give them a few days' extra life. It's not like a cooked preserve, more like the mint sauce served with Sunday lunch but with a kick for spicing up salads and savouries. This makes around 90ml/6 tablespoons worth.

Total calories: 26–38 for entire quantity
Preparation time: 5 minutes

> 25g herbs, such as coriander, mint, parsley, roughly torn, 6–18
> 1½ teaspoons ground cumin, 8
> ½–1 green chilli pepper, roughly chopped, 2–4
> Juice of ½ lemon or lime, 6
> *Optional: ¼ teaspoon of sugar or a few drops of agave nectar,*
> *4*

1. Put all the ingredients into the beaker of a stick blender/a tall jug. Push the herbs down and just cover with cold water.

2. Hand-blend until the herbs and pepper are well chopped and mixed: taste and add additional spices or sugar if required. Pour into a clean sealable jar and keep covered in the fridge. Use within a week: drizzle over salads or use as a dipping sauce.

P. S. Try adding finely grated fresh ginger and/or crushed garlic.

PANEER/TOFU TIKKA MASALA, 301/245 calories

I've always been envious of my partner for his regular order of chicken tikka masala at our favourite Indian takeaway. Here's my version for veggies or vegans, with a lower-fat twist (the restaurant version contains *loads* of cream). Paneer is one of my favourite ingredients, it is a mild but versatile Indian cheese; the calories vary a lot depending on brand, so look for a lower-fat version (I used Savera), or use tofu. Homemade masala marinade is delicious and quick to make with a hand blender, but you could save time by buying a paste – again, calories vary.

Serves 2
Preparation time: 15 minutes
Cooking time: 6–8 minutes

   200g paneer, 348, or firm tofu, 230, diced
   1 onion, chopped, 38
   1 red pepper, deseeded and chopped into small chunks, 30
   100g tomatoes, roughly chopped, 20
   ½ teaspoon coconut oil, 21
   2 level tablespoons strained Greek yogurt, 29-40, or coconut
       yogurt, 55–195
   Chopped fresh coriander, to serve, 2

For the tikka masala paste, 47 calories per serving with lowest-cal vegan yogurt/57 with lowest-cal dairy yogurt

1 teaspoon each whole coriander and cumin seeds, 10

1 teaspoon each turmeric, cayenne pepper and garam masala, 15

2 garlic cloves, crushed or roughly chopped, 8

4cm piece fresh ginger, peeled and grated, 8

1 red chilli, deseeded and chopped, 4

2 tablespoons tomato purée, 20–46

50g strained full-fat Greek yogurt, 48–65, or coconut yogurt 28–98

1. Place all the paste ingredients in the beaker for a stick blender (or a tall jug: you don't want chilli or garlic in your eye). Blend together until the whole mix is thick and fragrant. If using ready-made paste, stir 3 tablespoons into the yogurt, adding a little extra turmeric and garam masala if you have them. Place the mixture in a sealed plastic container until needed.

2. Mix the paneer or tofu into the paste to coat. Let it marinate in the fridge for 1 hour or overnight if you have time.

3. Fry the onion, pepper and tomatoes in the coconut oil in a medium saucepan for 2 minutes. Now add the paneer/tofu and paste to the pan with 50ml water. Cook, stirring gently, for 4–5 minutes until the sauce thickens. Stir the last bit of yogurt through just before serving. Add the coriander as a garnish, or serve with cauliflower rice (page 202).

P. S. The second portion keeps in the fridge (but maybe padlock it in the meantime, it's that delicious). For a halloumi version, make the tikka paste and fry with the vegetables and tomato sauce. In a separate non-stick frying pan, fry 100g of reduced-fat halloumi (230 calories) in ½ teaspoon of oil, until browned on both sides. Add to the curry sauce and serve immediately – halloumi is salty so doesn't need extra seasoning.

JAVANESE TEMPEH KEBABS WITH SWEET SOY MARINADE, 323 calories

Two ingredients that might be new for you here, both from Indonesia, but I promise they're worth trying. Tempeh is made from fermented soya beans – it comes in blocks like tofu but has a nutty taste and a satisfyingly chewy texture: nutritionally it's also high in protein, and the fermentation makes the nutrients more available to the body. Ketjap manis is a thick, Indonesian, sweetened soy sauce, and if you love balsamic vinegar or pomegranate molasses, it offers a similar sweet-sour kick. If you can't get hold of it, you could improvise with soy sauce and a little brown sugar, honey or agave mixed in.

Serves 1
Preparation time: 8 minutes (plus 1 hour for marinating)
Cooking time: 10 minutes

For the marinade

  2 teaspoons ketjap manis, 30
  2cm piece fresh ginger, peeled, 4
  1 garlic clove, 8
  ½ red chilli, finely chopped, 2

For the kebabs

  100g tempeh, cut into 9–10 cubes,190
  75g button mushrooms, 12
  ½ small courgette, cut into chunks, 17

½ teaspoon coconut or rapeseed/groundnut oil, 21

30g tinned or very fresh beansprouts, 9 (see important safety note below)

5g crushed peanuts, 28

Chopped coriander leaves, to garnish, 2

2-3 wooden or metal kebab skewers

1. If using wooden skewers, soak them in water so they don't burn when grilling.

2. For the marinade, place the ketjap manis into a small bowl and grate the garlic and ginger over, so you catch any liquid. Add the chopped chilli. Put the tempeh into the bowl and turn the pieces over so they're coated in the marinade. Leave for at least 1 hour to marinate.

3. Place the mushrooms and courgette chunks on the skewers, alternating them with the marinated tempeh.

4. To cook on a griddle, melt a little oil over a high heat then add the kebabs. Let the tempeh and veggies brown, then turn and continue cooking; repeat so that each side of the cubes are cooked.

5. Serve with very well-rinsed tinned or fresh beansprouts topped with the crushed nuts and chopped coriander.

Important: see safety note regarding beansprouts, page 93.

P. S. You can use the same marinade with tofu (from 115 calories per 100g). Also, try adding red pepper chunks or broccoli florets to the kebabs.

CAULIFLOWER RICE, 25 calories

Cauli rice is the ideal accompaniment to curries and stews that you'd usually soak up with rice. It's quick to make and much lower in calories than normal rice, plus it counts as one of your '5 a day' vegetable portions. It tastes much milder than you'd expect, too.

Serves 2
Calories per serving: 25
Preparation and cooking time: 5–10 minutes

200g cauliflower florets, 50
Freshly ground sea salt and black pepper, to taste

1. Grate or finely chop the cauliflower florets until they resemble rice grains. The fastest way to do this is to pulse the cauliflower florets in a food processor, which gives a finer texture.

2. Place the cauliflower into a loosely covered microwaveable dish. Don't add water: there's already enough in the cauliflower to stop it drying out. Place in the microwave and cook on full power for 2 minutes. If you are only cooking one portion, reduce the time to 60 seconds. If you prefer, you can stir-fry the grated cauliflower. Add a splash of water or spray a saucepan with 1 Cal cooking spray to prevent the 'rice' sticking and set over a high heat. When hot, add the cauliflower and fry for 2–3 minutes, or until softened. If you are using spray, the rice may caramelise a little, adding a nutty flavour.

3. Season and serve immediately.

P.`S. Try adding herbs or spices either when processing the cauliflower or during cooking; try cumin, ginger, fresh chillies or dried chilli flakes, or fresh herbs such as parsley or basil – all taste good. You can also freeze individual portions, which generally won't take much longer to reheat than if it was freshly prepared.

CHAPTER SIX

Comfort

Fasting can be trickier during the colder months as we can feel the chills, but this section proves you can max out the comfort without maxing out the calories. Try the rich, melting cheese and tomato sauce in the aubergine parmigiana, the quick suppertime savoury noodles, or the tarte tatin with the sweetest tomatoes and onions. P.S.: Lots of these recipes freeze well so they're great for batch cooking (see page 334 for more tips).

RECIPES

5:2 Lives

SANNA'S VEGGIE FASTING REVOLUTION

'Less is more. Less is enough!'

Before: couldn't run, didn't feel like myself
After: energetic, healthier and a lot lighter

It was the start of 2016, and illustrator Sanna Mander was fed up.

'My weight was 13 stone 3lb (84kg), and I just didn't feel like myself. I was weak, and couldn't run – even to the bus! I also missed being able to buy good-looking clothes from "normal" shops.'

Sanna, who is 36 and lives in Helsinki, Finland, had tried intermittent fasting when it became popular in 2013. 'It seemed like a good way of life because of not being on a diet 24/7, and also for the health benefits. I started 5:2 then, and followed it successfully for a couple of months, but stopped when I got pregnant.'

In 2016, with three children aged two, six and seven, Sanna realised it was time to give it another go. 'I planned what, and where to eat that day. I am a foodie so I was just excited to choose meals suiting the calorie limit, still flavourful and nice!'

Sanna eats vegan food on Fast Days, to get the most from her calories: so, she might have a chilled gazpacho soup, or a big dish of courgettes, marinated in chipotle pepper and then sautéed. She really enjoys the challenge of using seasonal ingredients: 'Less can be more. I can enjoy all the things one can make from one ingredient, like cabbage – soup, coleslaw, kimchi and stew, that's lots of food for two Fast Days!'

And the results came quickly. 'I have lost 1 stone 8lb (10kg) in 7 months. I used to wear a EU size 44/46, now I'll fit into 40/42. Yesterday I bought a pair of stretchy jeans that were sized "S"!'

But the differences she has noticed in her health have been just as satisfying. 'I have more energy. I have cleaned and organised our home a lot! And I haven't been sick at all since I began. At all! No flu, no infections, no stomach flus, NOTHING!'

Sánna had been a vegetarian most of her adult life – and though her husband Jonathan occasionally eats meat, their children have been veggie since birth. Yet even though she's always been thoughtful about food, 5:2 has brought more changes in her attitude. 'I used to think I need to get as much out of every meal as I can – as if it was my "duty" to eat the biggest ice cream, or choose the most indulgent meal at a restaurant. Now I can respect my own limits and listen to my hunger levels. Less is more. Less is enough!'

Fast Day routine:

I don't eat breakfast. I have a bottle of sparkling water and a cup of coffee. For lunch on a Fast Day I have salad with vegetables, or soup. For dinner, I have salad, soup or sautéed vegetables, always vegan. I have some rice cakes for a snack if I need something to nibble on. On a Fast Day, I drink 2 or 3 bottles of sparkling water, 3 cups of coffee and 2 cups of tea.

The other 5 days?
I did count calories for 6 months. Now I eat normally on non-Fast Days, meaning carbs and treats too! It hasn't affected the weight loss. My appetite depends on many things; I seem to eat more if the weather is cold or if I'm stressed at work!

The veggie life:
I choose not to eat meat because of compassion for animals and because the meat industry is sick. Nowadays there are a lot of 'meat-replacing' products available, which makes vegetarian meal planning for the entire family easier. Being a strict vegetarian is difficult when there are so many hidden animal products, like gelatine in candy (and toothpaste!). But veggie fasting is very easy. Vegetables are naturally low in calories and there are so many ways to cook them.

Top tips:
I'd suggest people think of meals they already have that are low-cal, and to eat those on weekly basis – so soup/salad, etc.

Last word:
I can buy nice clothes again! There are nice clothes for over-weight people available online, but I want to stroll around in shops and try out different things. I feel like running, jumping and dancing!

YORKSHIRE PUDS WITH SAGE AND MUSTARD MUSHROOMS, 211 calories

I had this idea one cold January evening when I wanted something hearty with a bit of crunch but I didn't fancy bread. Yorkshire puds with a filling were the perfect solution, and these ones are light because of the egg but feel indulgent and are *so* quick to make. You can flavour them in so many ways: fresh chopped herbs or mustard powder are also delicious. I've given the recipe for 3 servings (of 2 puds each) as they freeze well (or you could cheat with ready-made frozen mini puds).

Serves 3
Preparation time: 5 minutes (plus resting time for the batter)
Cooking time: 15 minutes

For the Yorkshire puddings, makes 6, 44 calories each, (a serving is 2 puddings, 88 cals)

1 medium egg, 66
60ml semi-skimmed milk, 29
40g plain flour, 144
½–1 teaspoon mixed dried herbs, 3–5
½ teaspoon rapeseed oil, 21
Freshly ground sea salt and black pepper, to taste

For the sauce, 41–48 per serving

½ onion, chopped, 19
½ teaspoon rapeseed/groundnut, 21

100g mixed mushrooms, chopped into large chunks, 20–25

1 teaspoon wholegrain or Dijon mustard, 5–10

A few sprigs or a good pinch of fresh or dried herbs of your
choice (tarragon or chives are good), 2

50g peas or petit pois, 30-40

1 level tablespoon half-fat crème fraiche, 26

You will also need a 6-hole muffin tin

1. Mix the egg, milk and flour together and whisk very well to ensure there
are no lumps, then add the herbs and season well. Leave the batter to
stand for at least 30 minutes (or overnight in the fridge).

2. When you're ready to bake the puds, preheat the oven to
230°C/450°F/Gas mark 8. Use a pastry brush to apply the rapeseed oil
to 6 hollows in the muffin tin and place in the oven for 5 minutes to heat.

3. Take out the pre-heated tin and divide the batter between the holes. Bake
for 12–14 minutes until browned and cooked through.

4. Meanwhile, fry the onion in the oil for 2 minutes then add the
mushrooms and fry at a high temperature until they're browned and
slightly caramelised. Reduce the heat and add the mustard and herbs and
cook for 2 more minutes. Boil or microwave the peas, then add the crème
fraiche to the mushroom mix and warm through gently. Season, then pile
on top of the puds with the peas on the side.

P. S. To freeze the puds, wait until they're fully cooled then
place them in a freezer bag or box. Reheat at 200°C/400°F/
Gas mark 6 for 8 minutes or until crisped up. You can also use
shop-bought frozen Yorkshire puds, which start at about 40
cals per pudding.

SIMPLEST SOBA SUPPER NOODLES WITH MUSHROOM AND EGG, 263 calories

(📳)(🌿) (check label as some soba noodles are a mix of wheat and buckwheat)

This does what it says on the tin – it's simple and tasty and is garlic- and onion-free (unless you garnish it with a few spring onions!), so you will have sweet breath the next morning. The heat level depends entirely on your chilli... There's no need for very fancy mushrooms for this, even boring buttons will do the job. Fast, filling and great for supper, lunch or even brunch.

Serves 1
Preparation time: 5 minutes
Cooking time: 10 minutes

40g thin buckwheat noodles, 138
1 teaspoon sesame oil, 41
50g mushrooms, sliced, 10–12
1 egg, 66
½ red chilli, chopped, 2
1 teaspoon soy or tamari sauce, 3–10
1 teaspoon rice vinegar, 1
Freshly ground sea salt and black pepper, to taste
Optional, to serve: 1 small spring onion, snipped or chopped, 2

1. Cook the noodles according to the packet instructions. Make sure you rinse the buckwheat noodles after cooking as they can be starchy.

2. Heat the sesame oil and fry the mushrooms over a high heat for 2 minutes. Set aside.

3. Now fry the egg with the chopped chilli in the same pan and oil.

4. Drain and rinse the noodles, add back to the pan with the mushrooms, soy or tamari and rice vinegar. Reheat briefly then place in a bowl with the fried chilli egg on top. Season and serve with the green spring onion tops, if using.

P. S. Use whatever veg you have in the fridge – small and light mangetout or maybe cooked broccoli or cauli. Try some of the different kinds of noodles: sweet potato has a lovely colour. For a vegan version, just fry 50g tofu (57 calories) or 50g tempeh (95) with the mushrooms.

COURGETTI CARBONARA WITH ASPARAGUS, 247 calories

When I wrote my first 5:2 book, courgetti wasn't even a 'thing', but now it's hard to find a courgette that hasn't been spiralised. No wonder – noodles made from julienned courgette are low in calories and lighter to eat than dense pasta. On a Fast Day, that means you can indulge in richer sauces than you could normally 'afford' calorie-wise with pasta, without blowing the calorie 'budget'. This is a rich, cheesy carbonara-style sauce with asparagus that feels a real treat. The sauce can scramble slightly without the copious fat used in 'real' carbonara, but it still tastes amazing!

Serves 1
Preparation time: 3 minutes
Cooking time: 5–6 minutes

> 100g asparagus spears, 27
> 1 medium courgette, 34
> 1 egg, 66
> 20g Grana Padano cheese, finely grated, 78
> 1 teaspoon olive oil, 41
> Freshly ground salt and pepper, a few fresh basil leaves to
>   garnish, 1

1. Use a julienne peeler or spiraliser to cut the courgette into thin noodles. Pat with kitchen roll to drain away as much excess moisture as possible.

2. If the asparagus spears are thick, trim the ends, cut into chunks and cook in lightly salted water for around 4 minutes. If they're the fine kind, cut in half and cook for more like 2–3 minutes. Drain the veg.

3. Break the egg into a bowl and add 15g of the cheese. Whisk with a fork till well mixed and then season with black pepper. Warm a pasta bowl.

4. Fry the oil in a large non-stick frying pan over a very high heat and stir-fry the courgette noodles until they're just starting to brown (no more than 1 minute). You don't want them to go soggy or release water. Now add the cooked asparagus, mix through and remove the pan from the heat.

5. Pour the egg and cheese mix over the courgetti and quickly stir through till it forms a sauce, then pour into the warmed bowl: it may scramble a little, but that won't affect the taste.

6. Season and top with the remaining cheese.

P. S. Swap the asparagus for peas, broad beans or mangetout: you can also add a little smoked Cheddar in place of the Italian cheese. NB: because the egg is only cooked briefly, this recipe is not suitable for those advised to avoid raw eggs.

INDIVIDUAL TOMATO AND ONION TARTE TATIN, 225 calories

Oh my, this is one of my favourites: an upside-down tart of tomatoes and onions, caramelised with balsamic vinegar and with a layer of crunchy filo. I make these in those retro, white metal pie dishes. But you can quadruple the ingredients and make in a springform cake tin to serve to family or friends: it'll take 10–15 minutes longer to cook, check that the filo is fully browned and the veggies softened.

Serves 1
Preparation time: 5 minutes
Cooking time: 30 minutes

200g mixed tomatoes – plum, cherry and some green, if you have them, 40

10g butter, 72, or 10ml/2 teaspoons olive oil, 82

Good handful of rosemary or thyme sprigs, 5

1 tablespoon balsamic vinegar, 5–20

1 small red onion, 38

1 x 25g sheet filo pastry, around 70 (dairy-free if vegan)

Freshly ground sea salt and black pepper, to taste

20g rocket leaves, to serve, 5

1. Preheat the oven to 200°C/400°F/Gas mark 6.

2. Halve the smallest tomatoes and chop the larger tomatoes so they're roughly equal size with smaller ones and they all have one flat cut side

which can lie flush with the bottom of the tin. Place onion on its side and cut 5 or 6 slices right through, keeping the rings together.

3. Melt half the butter or oil in a heavy-based frying pan and add the herbs and balsamic vinegar. Add the onion slices, whole, and the tomatoes, cut side down. Cook gently for 5–7 minutes (smaller tomatoes take less time) until the vegetables have softened and are starting to caramelise.

4. Transfer the veg to a pie dish or fluted springform tart tin, again, cut side down. Season with salt and pepper. Tear the filo into 2–3 sheets that roughly match the size of the dish and place on top, tucking them in at the edges. Melt the remaining butter and brush it over the top of the filo with a pastry brush.

5. Bake for 10–15 minutes (again, it depends on the size of the tomatoes) until the pastry is golden brown.

6. Turn out by placing a plate on top of the tin and inverting it/loosening the base if you have used a springform tin. Sprinkle more herbs on top and serve with the rocket leaves on the side.

P. S. You can add goat's cheese (25g is 63–83 calories depending on the brand) between the tomato layer and filo before cooking to create a tart, creamy filling.

HERBED POLENTA CHIPS WITH CRISPY GARLIC BROCCOLI, 232 calories

Purple-sprouting or tender-stem broccoli deserves to be the star of the show, and this is one of my favourite ways to serve the long stalks: spicy, garlicky and delicious, with crunchy polenta 'chips' on the side. This is written for two because it makes sense to make a batch of the polenta chips and keep the others ready for when you want them.

Serves 2 (make polenta slices in advance and keep in fridge/ freezer ready to use)
Preparation time: 5 minutes
Cooking time: 15 minutes

For the chips, 155 calories per serving

300ml vegetable stock (use 1 teaspoon vegetable bouillon to save time), 12
75g quick-cook polenta, 272, plus a little extra for dusting
1 teaspoon dried mixed/Italian herbs, 5
½ teaspoon rapeseed/groundnut oil for frying chips, 21

For the broccoli, 77 calories per serving

240g purple sprouting or long-stemmed broccoli, tough leaves and stalks trimmed, 86 (15–16 stalks)
2 garlic cloves, cut into thin strips, 8
1 red chilli pepper, deseeded and cut into thin strips, 4

½ teaspoon rapeseed/groundnut oil for frying garlic dressing, 21
Freshly ground sea salt and black pepper, to taste
5g toasted pine nuts, 34, or 10g Grana Padano cheese, 39, to serve

1. Prepare the chips in advance. Bring the stock to the boil, whisk in the polenta a little at a time, stirring well. Stir until cooked, around 8 minutes, then add the mixed herbs and plenty of sea salt and black pepper. Line a small, square baking tin with foil and spoon the polenta into it, smoothing it and flattening it down. Leave to set for at least 30 minutes.

2. Steam the broccoli in a pan of boiling water for 4–5 minutes, until it still has a little bite to it. Drain and 'refresh' in cold water.

3. Cut the set polenta into chip shapes and sprinkle with a little extra cornmeal. Heat the oil in a frying pan and fry the chips until lightly browned, 3–4 minutes. Arrange on two plates and keep warm in the oven.

4. Heat the oil in a frying pan then fry the garlic and chilli very carefully until they crisp up but don't burn – they can turn instantly, so keep a very close eye on them. Remove with a slotted spoon, then add the broccoli to the empty pan to warm up again.

5. Arrange the broccoli on top of the chips, divide the garlic and chilli among them and finish with the pine nuts or cheese.

P. S. The chips are the perfect accompaniment to any savoury topping, try them with pasta sauces or the mushroom topping from the Yorkshire pud dish on page 209.

ONE-POT SPELT SPAGHETTI WITH PEAS, THYME AND WHITE WINE, 305 calories

Vegan version with nutritional yeast: 307
Veggie version with ricotta: 317

One-pot pasta became a 'thing' on the internet a couple of years back – and who *doesn't* want to save on washing-up? This dish is super-quick, simple and really tasty, made from mostly store-cupboard supplies. The vegan version makes use of nutritional yeast for the umami flavour, while veggies can use light ricotta. I like it with spelt spaghetti, which some people find easier to digest than white pasta, although it's not gluten-free.

Serves 1
Preparation time: 3 minutes
Cooking time: 11–12 minutes

2 garlic cloves, crushed, 8
Leaves from 3 stalks of thyme or lemon thyme, 1
1 teaspoon extra-virgin olive oil, 41
50ml white wine, 33
Juice and zest of ½ lemon, 8
200ml water
45g spelt spaghetti, 162
50g frozen petit pois, 35

For the topping
5g nutritional yeast, 17, or 20g ricotta, 27

1. In a medium saucepan, fry the crushed garlic and most of the thyme leaves gently for 2 minutes in the oil.

2. Now add the wine, lemon juice, water and pasta and bring the liquid to the boil.

3. Cook for 7 minutes, then add the petit pois, and cook for a further 2–3 minutes. Towards the end of the cooking time, if needed, add more water, a tablespoon at a time, to stop the pasta drying out: you want a little liquid left as sauce.

4. When the pasta is just cooked, place into a warm bowl, season and add the nutritional yeast or ricotta, plus the lemon zest and the remaining thyme leaves.

P. S. This is super-versatile, though I find it works best with spaghetti or tagliatelle, as pasta shapes can be stodgy. Choose herbs, vegetables and toppings to suit the season: fry leeks, onion, spring onion or celery with the oil and add chilli, rosemary or dried herbs. Cook the pasta with broad beans or diced vegetables such as peppers, courgettes or tomato. Add fresh herbs, breadcrumbs, pine nuts or Parmesan to serve.

RICH AUBERGINE PARMIGIANA, 273 calories

A classic, for good reason! I've cut down a little on oil and used lower-fat mozzarella, but otherwise, this is the real deal and a generous portion, too. Layers of tender aubergine, hot cheese and full-flavoured tomatoes. 'Proper' parmesan isn't veggie, but Grana Padano is, and it also tastes very similar and is usually cheaper! If this is the Mediterranean diet, bring it on...

Serves 4
Preparation time: 20 minutes
Cooking time: 35–40 minutes

2 teaspoons olive, rapeseed or groundnut oil, 82
2 medium aubergines, around 200g each, thinly sliced
    lengthwise, 80
1 onion, chopped, 38
3 garlic cloves, chopped, 12
3 x 400g tins chopped tomatoes, 240
1 teaspoon dried oregano or 1 tablespoon fresh, 5
2 teaspoons sugar, 30, or 1 teaspoon agave nectar, 17
3 tablespoons red wine vinegar, 11
2 x 125g reduced-fat/light packets of mozzarella, 420
Handful of basil leaves, 5
25g breadcrumbs, 92
20g Grana Padano, finely grated, 78
Freshly ground sea salt and black pepper, to taste

1. Preheat the oven to 200°C/400°F/Gas mark 6.

2. Heat a griddle, measure out 1 teaspoon of oil and apply a little to the pan with a pastry brush. Grill the aubergine slices in batches on both sides until softened and lightly marked, but not charred: use more of the measured oil as needed. Set the slices aside on kitchen roll to drain away excess oil.

3. While the aubergines are grilling, fry the onion and garlic in a large non-stick pan for 2–3 minutes in the other teaspoon of the oil. Add the tinned tomatoes, oregano, sugar and red wine vinegar and cook for 5–8 minutes, covered, until the sauce thickens.

4. Tear the mozzarella into small pieces with your fingers. Take a lasagne or roasting dish and spoon tomato sauce onto the bottom, then cover with slices of aubergine. Season, then add more tomato sauce, followed by basil leaves and pieces of mozzarella. Continue to layer in this way: aubergine and seasoning; tomato sauce and mozzarella, ending with a thick layer of tomato sauce on the top.

5. Mix together the breadcrumbs and cheese and scatter over the top of the parmigiana. Bake for 40 minutes, until the cheese topping is crisp. Serve with a green salad.

P. S. You can prepare in advance to the end of stage 4 and then refrigerate before adding the topping and then baking. For a gluten-free version, leave out the breadcrumbs but double the Grana Padano! Leftovers will keep in the fridge for a couple of days, just reheat in the microwave, but the dish doesn't freeze well.

ROASTED CAULIFLOWER STEAK ITALIAN-STYLE, 179 calories

Vegetarian version with cheese: 179
Vegan version with pine nuts: 172

This is simple but delicious: cauliflower 'steaks', roasted with onion and cheese or nuts until they're caramelised. To help calculate portions, a medium cauli weighing 650g untrimmed will give you 2 'steaks' of around 180g each, plus another 200g or so of florets: you can also reheat or serve the second portion in a salad or as a side vegetable on a non-fasting day.

Serves 2
Preparation time: 10 minutes
Cooking time: 40–45 minutes

1 medium cauliflower, turned into 2 x 180g 'steaks' plus 200g florets, 140
2 teaspoons rapeseed/groundnut oil, 82
1 small onion, quartered, 38
Leaves from 3–4 rosemary sprigs, 2
20g Grana Padano cheese, grated, 84, or 10g pine nuts, 70
Freshly ground sea salt and black pepper, to taste
2 lemon wedges, 10, plus a few herb leaves, such as basil or parsley, 2, to serve

1. Preheat the oven to 220°C/425°F/Gas mark 7.

2. Remove the outer leaves of the cauli, then turn it upside down so the stalk faces you. Using a large knife (a breadknife is ideal), cut the cauli all the way through the middle, then trim the outside edges of the two halves to create two flat 'steaks' 2–3cm thick, plus numerous florets. Trim any remaining leaves without cutting the stalk.

3. Pour the oil into a shallow baking dish and place the cauliflower steaks, extra florets and the onion in the dish. Turn the vegetables over so all the pieces have a little oil on both sides, then season very well with salt and pepper and sprinkle over the rosemary.

4. Roast for 20 minutes, then turn the steaks and vegetable pieces over. If the cauli and onion are going too dark – you're aiming for browned/caramelised but not burned – turn the oven down to 200°C/400°F/Gas mark 6.

5. Check again after 15–20 minutes – when all the edges of the vegetables are well browned and the thickest part of the cauliflower is tender, sprinkle the grated cheese over the cauli pieces, if using. Return to the oven for 5 minutes, for the cheese to melt, or dry-fry the pine nuts in a small pan until they're just starting to brown.

6. Serve immediately, with the pine nuts, if using, lemon wedges and herbs.

P. S. This is hearty and filling on its own, but it's also delicious served with butternut squash mash: use 200g butternut squash (80) for 2 people. When you turn the cauli, place the squash alongside and sprinkle with more rosemary leaves. When cooked, simply mash lightly with a fork before serving alongside the steaks.

SWEET POTATO AND BLACK BEAN CHILLI WITH SMOKED PAPRIKA CREAM/AVOCADO, 226 calories

Vegetarian version with crème fraiche: 226
Vegan version with avocado: 229

This is hearty, smoky and utterly delicious. My partner – who hates sweet potato – happily cleared the bowl and asked for seconds, which is always a good sign. For vegans, an avocado cream replaces dairy – both are equally fantastic. This is also ideal for freezing (without the topping).

Serves 4
Preparation time: 10 minutes
Cooking time: 23–30 minutes

- 1 dried chipotle pepper, 23, or chipotle paste to taste (1 teaspoon is around 8 cals)
- ½ small jar roasted red peppers in oil, around 85g, drained, 59
- 2 small red or white onions, chopped, 76
- 3 garlic cloves, chopped, 12
- 1 teaspoon coconut or rapeseed/groundnut oil, 41
- 2 teaspoons ground cumin, 10
- 2 small sweet potatoes, around 300g, peeled and cut into cubes, 270
- ½ teaspoon agave, 8, or honey, 10

1 drained 380g vacuum pack or 1 x 400g tin of black beans,
   216
1 x 400g tin chopped tomatoes, 80
Freshly ground sea salt and black pepper, to taste
½ teaspoon smoked paprika, 3
4 level tablespoons half-fat crème fraiche, 104, or 75g
   avocado, 117
A sprinkling of chopped coriander leaves, 1, to serve

1. Rehydrate the dried chipotle in water for a few minutes. When ready,
   scrape out the seeds and chop finely. Drain the peppers and wipe with
   kitchen roll to remove as much oil as possible, then cut into chunks.

2. Fry the onions and garlic in the oil with the chopped pepper and cumin for
   2–3 minutes. Add the chipotle (or paste if using), potatoes and agave/
   honey, and gently fry for 1 more minute. Now add the black beans and
   tomatoes. Bring to the boil, then simmer, covered, for 20–25 minutes
   until the sweet potatoes are tender. Add water if needed to stop the sauce
   burning. Taste, and season well with salt and pepper.

3. Mix together the paprika and crème fraiche, or mash the avocado with
   the paprika. To serve, add a spoonful of cream or avocado to the centre
   of the bowl and sprinkle over the chopped coriander.

P. S. You can vary the beans in the chilli; tinned green lentils
give a more delicate flavour, while kidney beans make a more
traditional-looking chilli.

SIMPLE TOMATO SAUCE, 38 calories

Great for serving with any of the grain or pasta dishes in this book. You can adapt the basic flavour with the suggestions below. It keeps in the fridge in a covered container for 3–4 days, or it freezes well.

Makes 3 side servings, 38 calories per serving
Preparation time: 5 minutes
Cooking time: 5 minutes

½ teaspoon rapeseed/groundnut oil, 21
1 garlic clove, or 1 shallot, finely chopped, 4
1 x 400g tin chopped tomatoes, 80, or 400g ripe tomatoes, roughly chopped, 80
Good pinch sugar or ½ teaspoon agave nectar, 8
Freshly ground sea salt and black pepper, to taste

1. Heat the oil in a medium pan and gently fry the garlic or shallot for 2 minutes.

2. Add the chopped tomatoes and the sugar to the pan. Increase the heat and cook for another 3 minutes, breaking the tomatoes up with a spatula. Season well and serve.

VARIATIONS

Mexican sauce, 40 calories per serving

1. Fry 1 finely chopped fresh jalapeño or 1 teaspoon chipotle pepper paste from a jar and a chopped spring onion with the garlic. Sprinkle over a few chopped coriander leaves when serving.

Hot Italian, 53 calories per serving

1. Use 3 garlic cloves instead of one, plus 1 chopped red pepper and a finely chopped chilli pepper/good pinch of dried chilli flakes. Cook these for 5 minutes before adding the chopped tomatoes. Add either 1 teaspoon of Italian dried herbs when you add the tinned tomatoes, or a small handful of chopped fresh oregano, basil or marjoram at the end.

Warming Spicy Indian, 54 calories per serving

1. Chop a small onion and fry in a pan with coconut oil for 2 minutes before adding the garlic and ½ teaspoon each of turmeric, ground cumin and ground coriander. Serve sprinkled with chopped coriander leaves.

CHAPTER SEVEN

Share

Fasting is not about hiding away with a lettuce leaf while your friends, family or partner tuck into a hearty meal. All the dishes in this section are super-sociable or perfect for a cosy dinner for two, and so good no one will notice you're fasting. Plenty of them are also good for freezing, or for keeping in the fridge for a second meal later in the week.

RECIPES

OPEN BUTTERNUT SQUASH LASAGNE WITH ALMOND VEGAN PESTO, 🎁🥕, 191

MUSHROOM AND YELLOW CHILLI QUINOTTO RISOTTO WITH WHITE WINE, 🎁🥕🌾, 275

KALE AND PAPRIKA FALAFEL WITH POMEGRANATE AND HARISSA DRIZZLE, 🎁🥕🌾, 152

SQUASH AND SAGE ROAST, WITH YELLOW PEPPERS AND TOMATO HORSERADISH SAUCE, 🎁🥕, 224

BBQ KUMARA AND BEETS WITH A CRUNCHY PISTACHIO DUKKAH TOPPING, 🎁🥕🌾, 215

PISTACHIO DUKKAH TOPPING, 🎁🥕🌾, 41

ROASTED FIELD MUSHROOMS WITH FARRO WHEAT AND KALE, 🎁🥕, 249

FIVE SPICE TOFU AND MUSHROOMS WITH CHINESE PANCAKES, 🎁🥕, 248

SWEET AND SOUR AUBERGINE CAPONATA WITH PEAR, 🎁🥕🌾, 130

GLUTEN-FREE CRISPY SOCCA PIZZA, 🎁🥕🌾, 191 plus toppings

MINI BEETROOT SLIDERS WITH SLAW, 🎁🥕🌾, 131

5:2 Lives

JANICE RENEWS HER VOWS, 3 STONE (19KG) LIGHTER

'I can't stress how much this has done for me in a totally positive way.'

Before: depressed by her weight, bugged by health problems
After: three stone lighter, way more confident

It was four months before Janice Godfrey was due to renew her wedding vows to Wayne, and she desperate. At 5 foot 5, she weighed 14 stone (90kg) – she and her husband had gained weight after they got together.

'I think contentment took over – we were eating out, drinking and cooking for one another. Eventually it all caught up with me. My weight depressed me – I could not go into "ordinary" clothes shops to buy things to wear. I lost some confidence. I felt unfit and sluggish. I am a very social person but I started fretting about what to wear and how I looked when I was going out.'

Janice also had a series of health problems – gallstones, an operation to remove her gallbladder, and a severe kidney infection.

In happier news, the arrival of a new grandson made Janice wish she could be more active. 'I wanted to be able to run and swim with him.'

The breakthrough came on holiday in Portugal. 'I was on my "hen trip" before renewing my vows and I heard two of my girlfriends discussing the 5:2. I don't know why but it struck a chord with me. I felt like it was my last chance to do something before my big day. I thought, surely I could be good for two days a week.'

Janice, who is 55 and lives in Belfast, Northern Ireland, started the very next week. 'I was excited and nervous. I didn't want to fail. I made sure I had water and chewing gum to hand. I worked out the calorific value of lots of things that I felt I would like to eat and I made sure I was organised. When I completed my first fast I was delighted. Every fast I got under my belt made me more determined to keep going.'

Rapid results helped her motivation. 'I couldn't believe it. I lost 2 stone (13kg) very quickly (in about 2 months) and the last stone not long after. I could take my jeans off without opening them. I was a size 20 on top and a 16 on the bottom (could probably have done with an 18 at times). I am now a 14 on top and a 12 on the bottom. I'm still busty but now I can dress in a flattering way.'

Soon, others were noticing too. 'People I work with were constantly telling me I looked amazing. It took quite a bit of getting used to. I had to learn to accept compliments graciously. My boss of 20 years has told everyone about the "New Jan".'

Legal secretary Janice has now started running, completing several 5K runs, 'To me, it is a miracle. I feel energised and my skin is much better. I feel good – I don't know when I was last at the doctor. I'm positive and enjoy life. I go on beach holidays with my girlfriends. I am no longer embarrassed to be seen in a swimsuit, nice clothes or shorts.'

Now Wayne has joined in, losing two and a half stone so far.

'5:2 has changed my attitude to food. I now recognise when I am full and don't feel the need to stuff myself or finish everything on my plate. Usually by dinner time on a Sunday night I am looking forward to my Monday fast. I feel that my body enjoys the rest from three square meals a day. On those days, I now look after my body in other ways – I'm really into face creams, body scrubs, creams, using fake tan, etc. – things I never had time for before. I think I'd just got so down about myself that I was neglecting myself.'

Fast Day routine:

I save my calories for dinner on Fast Days, I don't eat until approx. 6.30pm. That would be from about 7pm the previous evening – so quite a long stretch. During the day, I drink as much water as possible (usually fizzy) and I chew gum. For dinner, I don't eat much: for example, toasted bread with sliced tomato to make a tomato toastie. I also have a cup of tea, and at 9pm I have low-cal toast with a smear of marmalade. I think I do eat too much bread but I find this suits me.

The other 5 days:

I have never counted calories on non-Fast Days. I eat and drink whatever I want. I like curries, pasta, mushrooms, spinach, all veg really – one-dish meals that are easy to make on a busy weeknight. I believe that alcohol played as big a part in my

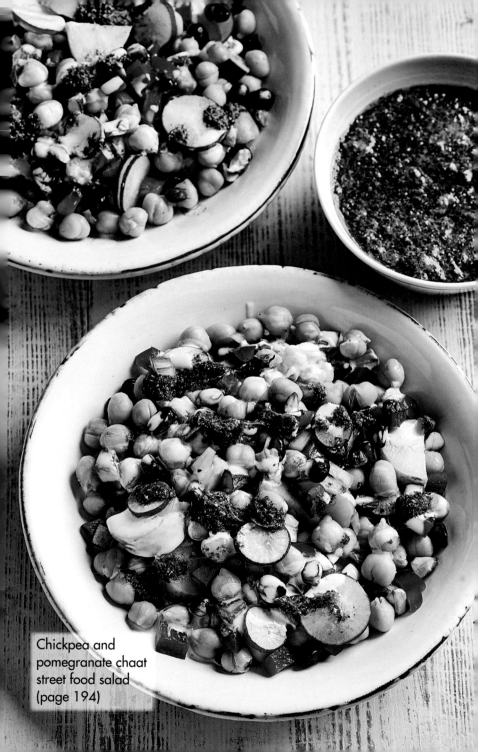

Chickpea and
pomegranate chaat
street food salad
(page 194)

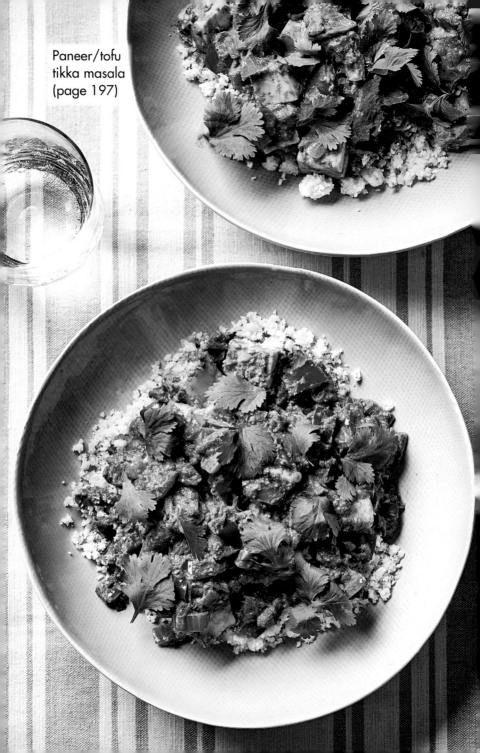

Paneer/tofu
tikka masala
(page 197)

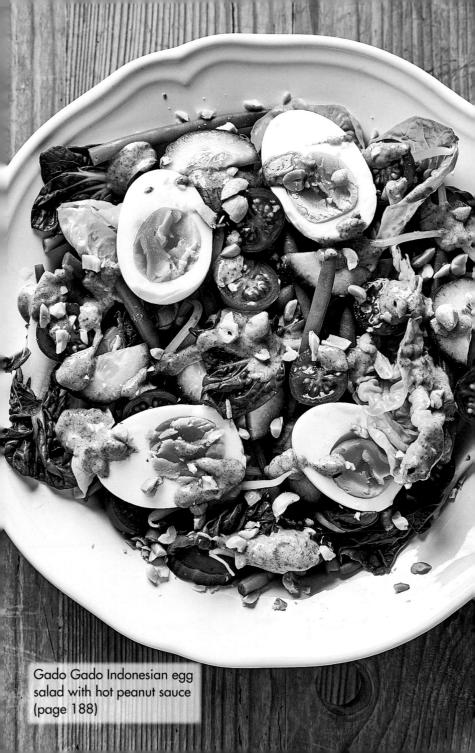

Gado Gado Indonesian egg
salad with hot peanut sauce
(page 188)

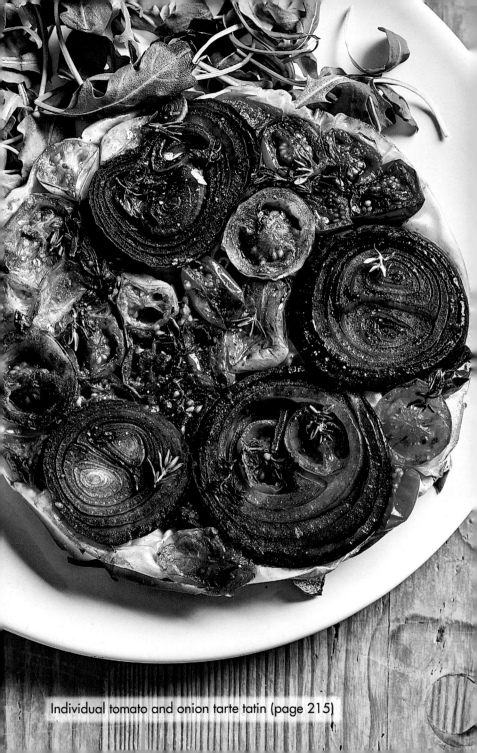

Individual tomato and onion tarte tatin (page 215)

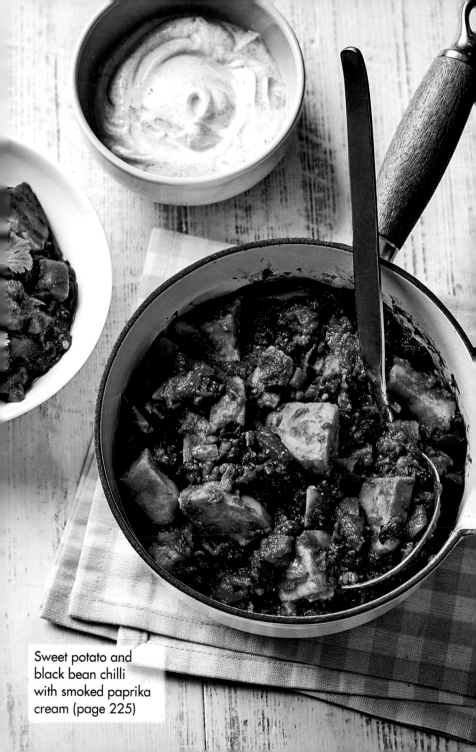

Sweet potato and
black bean chilli
with smoked paprika
cream (page 225)

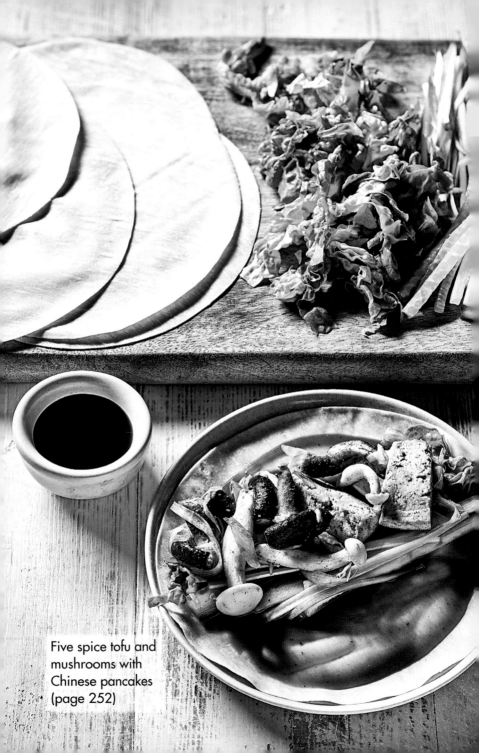

Five spice tofu and
mushrooms with
Chinese pancakes
(page 252)

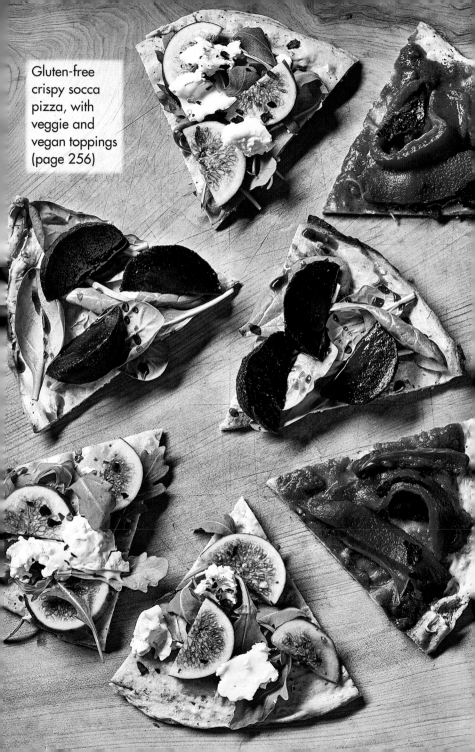

Gluten-free crispy socca pizza, with veggie and vegan toppings (page 256)

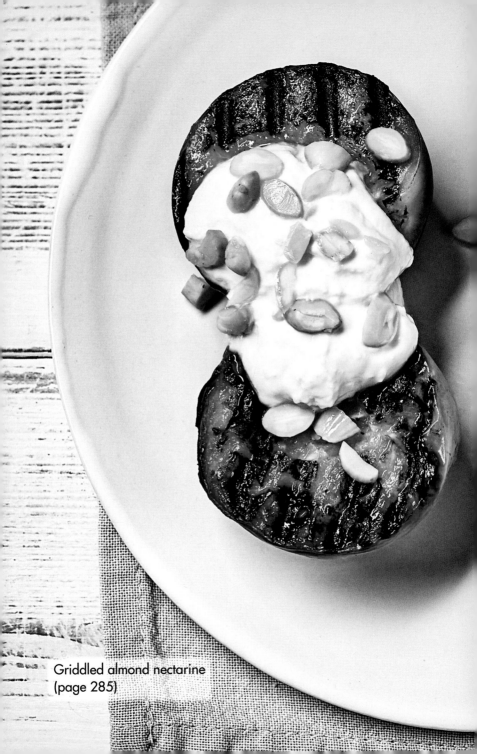

Griddled almond nectarine
(page 285)

weight gain as food. My husband and I had the very bad habit of having wine almost every night. Now I very rarely drink during the week.

The veggie life:

I became a vegetarian (or grass-eater as my six-year-old grandson calls me) on 1 January. For about a year before this I was eating less and less meat. I just didn't fancy eating it. 5:2 lends itself to being a veggie because vegetables are so low in calories. I've always loved vegetables anyway, so it's no hardship. I've been known to take a Sunday roast and just pass my hubby the meat. Last week I cooked a veggie wellington for my family and they all had a piece with their Sunday dinner.

Top tips:

Prepare mentally and food-wise, have healthy stuff around that you want to eat because otherwise you'll just open the fridge door and grab the first thing to stave off hunger. I also advise people to weigh themselves, measure themselves and to choose an item of clothing that is either a good fit or too tight in order to monitor their progress, and I also say take pics. Some people don't seem to lose weight, but they do lose inches.

Last word:

I want to enjoy my life as much as possible and I feel 5:2 has had a massive impact on me. I can't stress how much this has done for me in a totally positive way.

OPEN BUTTERNUT SQUASH LASAGNE WITH ALMOND VEGAN PESTO, 191 calories

(🍲)(🥕)(🌾) if using gluten-free pasta
Vegan version: 193
Vegetarian version with ricotta: 227

When I first became a veggie, the best you could hope for when eating out was a factory-made frozen veggie lasagne. That's probably why I rarely make the traditional kind at home. But I do like open lasagne which looks appealing and feels less stodgy. This version uses one small sheet of pasta per person, sandwiched around a purée of butternut squash and chilli, and a fantastic vegan pesto. If you eat dairy, you may want to add a little ricotta cheese, too.

Serves 2
Preparation time: 10 minutes
Cooking time: 25 minutes total

> 250g butternut squash, peeled and cut into chunks, 100
> A pinch of chilli flakes or Italian herbs, 1
> 2 dry whole-wheat or spinach lasagne sheets, 34g, 116, or
>   80g fresh, 128
> 1 teaspoon nutritional yeast, 17
> *Optional: 50g ricotta cheese, 68*

For the pesto sauce, 74 calories per serving

> Good handful/5g basil leaves, 5
> 2 garlic cloves, 8

2 tablespoons tomato purée, 20–46
1 teaspoon olive oil, 41
10g almonds, 58
Juice and zest of 1 lemon, 15
Freshly ground sea salt and black pepper, to taste

1. Place the squash in a saucepan and just cover with water. Add a good pinch of chilli flakes or Italian herbs and bring the water to a simmer. Cook for around 20 minutes, topping up the water if needed, until the squash has softened. Drain off as much water as possible then mash with a spatula or fork.

2. Meanwhile, make the pesto by either processing all the ingredients together in a mini-processor or by chopping the garlic roughly before pounding together all the other ingredients in a pestle and mortar.

3. Cook the lasagne sheets according to the packet instructions until al dente: most fresh will take 4–5 minutes, dried pasta 8–10.

4. Preheat the oven to 150°C/300°F/Gas mark 2. Assemble the lasagne on two ovenproof serving plates. Cut the lasagne into six oblong pieces. Place the first piece on the plate, then add a layer of squash purée and a layer of pesto, plus ricotta, if using. Add the next layer of pasta, like making a sandwich, and repeat the layer of squash/pesto, before adding the last sheet and topping with the squash, pesto and a good sprinkling of nutritional yeast. Repeat on the other plate.

5. Now let the lasagne reheat in the oven for 5 minutes. Season and serve.

P. S: For a different version, use the caponata from page 254as a filling, with the pesto or a little grated cheese between the layers.

237

Extra garnish: Serve with fried sage leaves for an extra delicious twist. Heat ½ teaspoon olive oil or butter (18–21 calories) in a small non-stick pan and add 5 or 6 fresh sage leaves: fry very gently until crispy but not blackened. Drain on kitchen towel then sprinkle over the top of the pasta.

MUSHROOM AND YELLOW CHILLI QUINOTTO RISOTTO WITH WHITE WINE, 275 calories

Vegan version: 275
Vegetarian version with crème fraiche or cheese: 301/295

There's nothing as comforting as risotto but for a change, I like to use other grains. High in protein and gluten-free, quinoa is actually a kind of seed, but it works well here. It can be bland, so I've pepped it up with a sauce made from the Peruvian 'aji amarillo' yellow chilli which has a delicious hot and fruity flavour. But this works well with other hot chilli sauces, too: use as much as you can handle. Do rinse quinoa very well in a fine-mesh sieve before cooking, to remove the natural coating which can add a soapy taste. Or to make this super-quick, use quinoa from a pre-cooked pack (you can keep the rest of the pack refrigerated and use it the next day).

Serves 2
Preparation time: 10 minutes
Cooking time: 23–28 minutes

80g quinoa, 292, or 180g pre-cooked quinoa, 320
2 teaspoons truffle oil, 82, or 5g butter, 72
250g mushrooms, such as chestnut, oyster, shiitake, sliced, 62
2 garlic cloves, chopped, 8
2 long shallots, peeled and chopped, around 60g, 14
1 small green chilli, chopped, 4

2 yellow or orange peppers, deseeded and sliced, 60

100ml white wine or vegetable stock, 66/24

1–2 teaspoons hot chilli sauce, ideally aji amarillo, 4–8

50g baby spinach or mixed spinach, rocket and watercress, 12

Optional: 2 level tablespoons half-fat crème fraiche, 52, or

10g Grana Padano cheese, 40

1. Rinse the quinoa well, cover with water and then simmer according to the packet instructions (usually 20–25 minutes): check regularly and top up with water if the quinoa dries out before it's cooked. Drain once ready.

2. Heat half the oil or butter in a large non-stick pan and fry the mushrooms on high, letting them brown. After 2–3 minutes, reduce the heat and add the garlic, shallots, chopped chilli and peppers. Fry for 3 more minutes, then add the stock or wine and the hot chilli sauce. Cook for 3 more minutes, until the liquid reduces. Now stir through the cooked quinoa and green leaves, and let them warm through.

3. Season well, place in a serving dish and dot with the remaining oil or butter. Stir in the crème fraiche or grate over the cheese, if using.

P. S. If you are serving one, you can keep the second portion in the fridge and reheat gently (don't add the crème fraiche or cheese until serving). Vary the vegetables and flavours – try it with fresh broad beans, leeks and asparagus, with a garnish of tiny fresh mint leaves.

KALE AND PAPRIKA FALAFEL WITH POMEGRANATE AND HARISSA DRIZZLE, 152 calories

This recipe has been the trickiest in the book to perfect – but it's been worth it! When you buy falafel from a stall, fresh-fried, it gets a lot of its texture from the hot oil. Creating a great-tasting lower-calorie version means adding *loads* of extra flavours: savoury kale, garlic, warming paprika, leafy herbs and nutty tahini – plus a fruity, spicy dip. Baking these falafel means they have a softer texture than the traditional fried version, but they are much more fast-friendly.

Serves 4 (4 falafel per person), 128 per serving
Preparation time: 10 minutes
Cooking time: 20 minutes

75g kale, 30
1 x 400g tin chickpeas, drained, 312
2 garlic cloves, 8
1 teaspoon ground paprika, 5
1 teaspoon ground cumin or ras al hanout, 5
20g/1 pack coriander and/or parsley leaves, 7
5 spring onions, roughly chopped, 10–15
2 teaspoons tahini, 60
1 teaspoon rapeseed/groundnut oil, 41
5g sesame seeds, 32
Freshly ground sea salt and black pepper, to taste

To serve

1 tablespoon pomegranate molasses, 40

1 tablespoon water

¼ teaspoon harissa or dried chilli flakes, 3–5

2 Little Gem lettuces, leaves separated, 30

1 lemon, cut into quarters, 12

1 tablespoon pomegranate seeds, 12

1. Preheat the oven to 200°C/400°F/Gas mark 6. Wash and carefully dry the kale, and remove any very thick stems. Process well on their own in a food processor.

2. Add the drained chickpeas, garlic, ground spices, herbs, plus half the spring onions and half the tahini. Process well until the mixture comes together. Test with a teaspoon – the mix should be dough-like but not too dry: add the extra tahini if needed. Add plenty of sea salt and pepper to taste, and stir through the rest of the spring onions.

3. Line a baking tray with non-stick baking paper. Take a dessertspoonful of the mix at a time and shape into oval patties with your hands: there should be enough for 16 small falafels. Place on the baking tray and, using a pastry brush, brush the oil across the tops of the falafel, followed by a sprinkling of the sesame seeds.

4. Bake for 20 minutes until the outsides are browned. Meanwhile, whisk together the molasses, water and harissa or dried chilli flakes. Arrange the lettuce leaves on four plates with the lemon wedges, and when the falafels are cooked, scatter over the pomegranate seeds and serve with the molasses mix as a drizzle or a dip.

P. S. Try different spices in the mix – cayenne pepper, whole cumin or coriander will all work. You can keep the mix in the fridge, uncooked but covered, for up to 3 days, or freeze after baking, with layers of greaseproof paper between them. Defrost and then reheat in the microwave or oven.

SQUASH AND SAGE ROAST, WITH YELLOW PEPPERS AND TOMATO HORSERADISH SAUCE, 224 calories

This is perfect for a family get-together and the leftovers fit the bill for a Monday Fast Day. The loaf is moist and full of good grains, and the colourful, spicy sauce and yellow peppers make it look lovely as a centrepiece. It takes a while to make but most of the cooking time is hands-off.

Serves 6 with 2 slices each. Calories per serving 224
Preparation time: 15 minutes
Cooking time: 1 hour 15 minutes

    100g quinoa, 365
    100g pearl barley, 352
    Flesh from 1 small coquina squash, peeled and cut into 1cm
        thick slices, 80
    2 yellow peppers, deseeded and sliced, 60
    4 garlic cloves, 16
    1 x 400g tin kidney beans, drained, 300
    50g cooked chestnuts, chopped, 80
    1 bunch of sage leaves, finely chopped, 10
    2 teaspoons salt
    Freshly ground sea salt and black pepper, to taste

For the sauce, 14 per serving

    ½ x 400g tin chopped tomatoes, 40
    Juice of 1 lemon, 12

1 teaspoon horseradish sauce, 30 (check label as horseradish
    cream is not vegan)

1. Cook the quinoa and pearl barley in a pan of boiling water with 1
   teaspoon of salt according to the packet instructions. While this is
   cooking, line a 2lb/950g loaf tin with non-stick paper. Preheat the oven
   to 190°C/375°F/Gas mark 5.

2. Place the squash slices and peppers on a tray lined with non-stick paper
   with the garlic cloves and season with a pinch of salt and pepper. Cover
   with foil and bake in the oven for 30–35 minutes until soft.

3. Once cooked, remove the garlic skins and blend together the squash,
   garlic and drained kidney beans. Set aside the peppers for later. Mix
   with the drained cooked quinoa, pearl barley and most of the chopped
   chestnuts, reserving a few for the tops. Stir the sage through the mixture.
   Press the mixture into the loaf tin and sprinkle with a few uncooked
   grains of quinoa, chestnuts and a pinch of salt. Cover with foil.

4. Bake in the oven for 30 minutes, then remove the foil and cook for a
   further 15 minutes or until the edges are just turning brown and crispy.

5. Remove from the oven and allow to cool in the tin before removing and
   slicing into portions.

6. To make the sauce, mix all the ingredients together in a small pan and
   heat gently, taste to check seasoning.

7. Serve with a few slices of the roasted pepper and a spoonful of sauce.

P. S. If you're not a fan of sage, parsley would work just as well.
Try toasting the slices for extra texture the next day – pop the
slices in the toaster, or if they crumble too much, do them

under the grill. Reheat in the oven or microwave.

This will keep and freeze well: freeze in portions and defrost slowly, then reheat in the oven or microwave.

BBQ KUMARA AND BEETS WITH A CRUNCHY PISTACHIO DUKKAH TOPPING, 215 calories

This combination of homemade dukkah spice mix, kumara (the name used in New Zealand for orange sweet potatoes) and beetroot makes for a colourful dish that works on the barbie, or on a grill pan if the weather isn't cricket.

Serves 2
Preparation time: 10 minutes
Cooking time: 10 + 6 minutes

> 1 sweet potato, around 200g, 180
> 1 pack of vacuum-packed beetroot in water (not in brine), 106
> Juice of 1 lime or lemon, 12
> 1 teaspoon rapeseed/groundnut oil, 41
> 2 servings dukkah, 90 (see next page for recipe)

1. Place the unpeeled potato in a pan of water, bring to the boil and cook until the potato is just tender but still firm, 10–12 minutes. When cool, slice into long thin wedges or chips.

2. Remove the beetroot from the packet and rinse briefly, then cut into wedges or halves depending on the size of the beetroot.

3. Mix the lemon or lime juice with the oil. Heat the griddle or barbecue and use a pastry brush to apply the juice and oil to both sides of the potato. Griddle or barbecue until the chips are softer and have clear grill marks, around 3 minutes, then turn over and cook on the other side. Do the

same with the beetroot — this will take less time, around 2 minutes on each side.

4. When the veggies are cooked, arrange them on a plate, pour over the cooking juices from the pan and sprinkle the dukkah on top. Eat warm!

P. S. This dish also works well with orange juice in place of the lime/lemon, and the addition of a dollop of crème fraiche or coconut yogurt.

PISTACHIO DUKKAH TOPPING, 41 calories

Dukkah is an Egyptian blend of whole nuts, seeds and spices, but I saw it used in lots of dishes when I was eating out in Australia. It's easy to make your own, just toast the whole spices and nuts in a pan, then grind them in a pestle and mortar or coffee grinder. Nuts are nutritious but high in fat, so a little goes a long way: this amount gives 4 servings, and you can keep the rest in an airtight container.

Makes 4 servings

½ teaspoon cumin seeds, 5
½ teaspoon coriander seeds, 5
½ teaspoon black mustard seeds, 5
10g sesame seeds, 61
15g unsalted pistachios, 89

1. Toast the whole spices, sesame seeds and pistachios in a non-stick frying pan. Be careful, as they can burn very quickly.

2. When they're browned, tip into a pestle and mortar or coffee grinder, and grind into a crunchy mix.

ROASTED FIELD MUSHROOMS WITH FARRO WHEAT AND KALE, 249 calories

The smell of mushrooms roasting in garlic and lemon will fill your kitchen when you make this – it's great for a shared supper, as well as an easy night in. Like the salad on page 154, it uses farro or emmer wheat: these are not suitable for coeliacs (see the P.S. for alternatives). If you only need one portion, use what's left over to stuff pepper halves the next day.

Serves 2
Preparation time: 5 minutes
Cooking time: 15 minutes

2 garlic cloves, crushed, 8
1 teaspoon rapeseed/groundnut oil, 41
Juice and zest of 1 lemon, 12
300g Portobello or field mushrooms (3–4), 74
A few thyme sprigs, 2
75g quick-cook farro, 271
1 bay leaf, 0
50g young kale, chopped and hard stalks removed, 20
10g pine nuts, toasted, 70
Freshly ground sea salt and black pepper, to taste
Optional: 25g melting cheese such as dolcelatte or brie, thinly sliced, 61–80

1. Preheat the oven to 200°C/400°F/Gas mark 6. Mix the garlic with the oil and lemon juice (retain the lemon zest).

2. Line a baking tray with foil, turning up the edges to collect the cooking juices. Place the mushrooms, gills up, and pour over the lemon, garlic and oil mix, top with the thyme sprigs, then roast in the oven for 15 minutes.

3. Add the farro and bay leaf to a pan with enough boiling water to cover. Simmer for 10–12 minutes until all the water has been absorbed, adding a little more water if it dries out (or follow the pack instructions). When cooked, stir through the kale to wilt.

4. Remove the mushrooms from the oven and cut into quarters. Add the mushrooms and the juices to the cooked farro. Season well and sprinkle over the lemon zest and pine nuts. If you're using cheese, slice it very thinly and tuck it under the hot farro so the cheese melts into the mix.

P. S. Use cavolo nero or chard in place of kale, or try roasting red and yellow peppers with oregano using the same method, removing the stalks and seeds and then roasting the halves in the oil mix. If you prefer a gluten-free dish, the mushrooms are also delicious served with cooked quinoa or puy lentils.

FIVE SPICE TOFU AND MUSHROOMS WITH CHINESE PANCAKES, 248 calories

(ⓘ)(✐)(🌾) – if not using pancakes

Fun to share, and utterly delicious, these are the vegan equivalent of Chinese crispy duck pancakes, with an appetising tofu and mushroom filling. Marinate in advance, then it's so quick to whip up.

Serves 2
Preparation time: 10 minutes plus 1+ hour marinating
Cooking time: 6–8 minutes

2cm piece fresh ginger, peeled and grated, 4
1 tablespoon tamari or soy sauce, 9–30
2 tablespoons rice wine vinegar, 6–10
1 teaspoon five spice powder, 5
100g exotic mushrooms, such as shiitake, oyster, cut into chunks, 20–25
100g tofu, cut into chunks, 115
1 small leek, around 100g, sliced lengthwise, 30
1 teaspoon sesame oil, 21
½ teaspoon agave nectar, 8, or honey, 10
6 Chinese pancakes, 204, or whole leaves of 1 Little Gem lettuce, 15
½ small cucumber, sliced into thin strips, 14
4 spring onions, sliced into thin strips, 8
30g lettuce, shredded, 5
20ml ready-made hoisin sauce, 45

1. Mix the grated ginger with the tamari or soy, vinegar and five spice powder in a bowl, adding the mushrooms and tofu (if there's not quite enough liquid, add a tablespoon of water). Marinate for at least 1 hour, or overnight in fridge.

2. Fry the leek for 2–3 minutes in sesame oil until it softens and browns a little. Add the marinated tofu and mushrooms and cook for another 3–4 minutes. Add the agave or honey and cook for a further minute.

3. Meanwhile, heat the pancakes according to the packet instructions, if using.

4. Serve the pancakes and mushroom mix at the table with the cucumber, spring onions, lettuce and sauce in little bowls. Spread each pancake with sauce, add the mushroom/tofu mix, top with salad and enjoy!

P. S. To bring the calories right down, use Little Gem lettuce leaves instead of pancakes, which makes it just 152 calories per serving. Try using tempeh (190 calories per 100g) in place of tofu, and roasted peppers instead of mushrooms.

SWEET AND SOUR AUBERGINE CAPONATA WITH PEAR, 130 calories (147 with pine nuts)

Slow-cooked aubergine and tomato-based dishes sum up the Med for me: French ratatouille, Catalan escalivada and this, Sicilian caponata. I love the sweet-sour taste delivered by the capers, vinegar and a little sugar (you can leave this out if you prefer). Plus, a secret ingredient here – discovered in Viana La Place's brilliant book, *Verdura* – is a pear! Add more or fewer capers to taste. This is wonderful on its own, or with a little sourdough or ciabatta bread or some radicchio. It keeps for several days in the fridge, and the flavours will mellow and intensify. It's best eaten warm or at room temperature, so take it out of the fridge before serving.

Serves 4
Preparation time: 10 minutes
Cooking time: 40–45 minutes

    4 teaspoons olive oil, 164
    1 medium aubergine, 300g, cut into 2cm cubes, 60
    1 medium courgette, cut into 2cm cubes, 34
    1 onion, roughly chopped, 38
    1–2 celery sticks, sliced into 2cm pieces, 12
    1 small pear, roughly chopped, 50
    1 x 400g tin chopped Italian tomatoes, 80
    1–2 tablespoons capers, roughly chopped, 11
    30g green olives, pitted and roughly chopped, 30

2 teaspoons sugar or 1 teaspoon agave nectar, 30, or honey, 15

4 tablespoons red wine vinegar, 12

Freshly ground sea salt and black pepper, to taste

Good handful fresh flat leaf parsley, 5, or 10g pine nuts, 70, to serve

1. Heat 2 teaspoons of the oil in a large non-stick saucepan and fry the aubergines over a medium heat for 8–10 minutes, until softened and lightly browned. Transfer to kitchen roll while you cook the courgette in another teaspoon of oil. Fry for 5–7 minutes until browned, then place on kitchen roll.

2. Meanwhile, heat 1 more teaspoon of oil in the same pan, add the onion, celery and a sprinkling of salt and fry gently for 5 minutes until the vegetables are soft. Add the pear, tomatoes, capers, olives, sugar/nectar and vinegar and cook for 10–15 minutes until it turns into a thick sauce. Now add the aubergines and courgettes and cook for 5 more minutes.

3. Before serving, season well and stir in the parsley or top with the pine nuts.

P. S. There are many variations on this recipe, chilli flakes are an authentic Sicilian addition, while a few raisins – high in sugar, so not too many – will add more sweetness to the dish.

GLUTEN-FREE CRISPY SOCCA PIZZA, WITH VEGGIE AND VEGAN TOPPINGS, 191 calories plus toppings 40–83 calories

Gluten-free pizza can be fiddly – but not this one. This version is made from chickpea/gram flour, which has been used in France and Italy for centuries to make 'socca' or 'farinata' pancakes. It's crispier than wheat pizza, and works with an infinite number of toppings. I especially love them with uncooked veg and salad, which complement the crispy base perfectly.

Makes 1 pizza base to serve 2, 191 per half
Preparation time: 5 minutes
Cooking time: 6–8 minutes

> 100g chickpea/gram flour, 336
> Good pinch of salt
> 1 tablespoon fresh herbs, finely chopped, such as thyme,
>   oregano, rosemary, or 1 teaspoon dried herbs, 5
> 100ml water
> 1 teaspoon rapeseed/groundnut oil, 41

1. Place the flour, salt and chopped or dried herbs in a bowl and combine. Add the water a little at a time and whisk in to create a thick, smooth batter. Leave to stand for at least 20 minutes.

2. Preheat the grill to high and place a pizza-sized square of greaseproof or baking paper on a baking tray. Using a large non-stick frying pan,

heat the oil, then pour the batter into the pan, tipping the pan to ensure it's evenly distributed. Cook for 3 minutes on a medium heat, until the underside is lightly browned and the top is beginning to set.

3. Use a spatula to transfer the pizza base to the baking sheet, cooked side down. Place under the grill for 3–5 minutes until the top is browned. If you're planning to use hot toppings, add those once the top is lightly browned and return to the grill. If not, add cold toppings and serve immediately – socca pizza tastes best fresh.

Toppings (per pizza to serve 2)

A socca pizza is a fantastic blank canvas for your favourite toppings. Here are a few of my suggestions (invent your own and tot up the calories using the chart on page 344).

Vegan

2 tablespoons of sun-dried tomato purée (20–40) with 2 roasted peppers from a jar, drained and sliced (60) – 40–50 calories per serving.

2 cooked beetroots (53), 20g baby spinach leaves (5) and 1 dessertspoon balsamic glaze or pomegranate molasses (26) – 42 calories per serving.

Thin layer of chilli jam (around 2 teaspoons, 38) with 15g rocket (4), 10g toasted pine nuts (70) and 16g sun-dried tomatoes, well drained and sliced (32) – 72 calories per serving.

Veggie

50g ricotta cheese (68) with 100g lightly cooked or roasted asparagus (27), sea salt flakes and zest of 1 lemon (3) – 49 calories per serving.

25g crumbled goat's cheese (63), 1 sliced fig (43), good pinch of chilli flakes (2), 15g rocket leaves (4) – 56 calories per serving.

100g thinly sliced ripe tomatoes (20), ½ ball reduced-fat buffalo mozzarella (100) and 2 peppadew peppers, thinly sliced (45) – 83 calories per serving.

P. S. You can use the same mix to make 2 individual pizzas in an omelette pan. Socca is best eaten when freshly cooked but you can pop it under the grill to reheat – the microwave will make it turn soggy.

MINI BEETROOT SLIDERS WITH SLAW, 131 calories per person

(🍱)(🥕)(🌾) (ensure oats are labelled as prepared in a gluten-free factory)

These are such fun for a party or to feed a crowd. If you've ever seen those bite-sized burgers served in cool bars and fancied a veggie version, these are for you. The mini-burgers are spicy and filling, and serving them using mushrooms as 'buns' makes them gluten-free and adds another veggie to this nutrient-rich meal. The simple slaw is super-colourful too.

Serves 8 (2 sliders each plus slaw)
Preparation time: 10 minutes
Cooking time: 15–20 minutes

For the sliders, 96 calories per person

50ml boiling water, 0
50g oats, 178
3 raw beetroot, peeled, 84
1 shallot, chopped, 2
1 jalapeño chilli, 6
1 x 400g tin kidney beans, drained, 300
16 Portobellini mushrooms, stalks removed, 600–700g, 160
1 large tomato, finely sliced, 20
Few lettuce leaves, 5
Gherkin slices, 10
Freshly ground sea salt and black pepper, to taste

For the slaw, 35 per portion

15g mixed seeds, 90
½ small white cabbage, around 300g, finely shredded, 72
Handful of coriander leaves, 5
50g sweetcorn, 45
50g pomegranate seeds, 50
1 red chilli, sliced, 4
Juice of 1 lime, 12

1. Preheat the oven to 180°C/350°F/Gas mark 4. Line 2 baking trays with non-stick paper. Pour the boiling water over the oats and leave to soak for 5 minutes.

2. In a food processor, blitz two of the beetroots with the shallot, chilli and the kidney beans until just smooth. Dice the remaining beetroot and mix through along with the oats and a pinch of salt and pepper.

3. Shape the mix into 16 small patties (each using 1 tablespoon of mixture) and place on the lined tray, along with the mushrooms. Drizzle a little water over the mushrooms and season with salt and pepper. Bake in the oven for 15 minutes. Check the mushrooms and burgers are cooked, if not, they may need a further 5 minutes.

4. While the burgers are cooking, make the slaw. Toast the seeds in a dry frying pan until they begin to pop. Mix with all the remaining slaw ingredients in a large bowl, with a pinch of salt and pepper. Leave to marinate while the burgers finish cooking.

5. Once everything is ready, build your burgers with the beetroot between two mushrooms. Add tomato slices, gherkins, whatever takes your fancy.

P. S. To freeze, bake the sliders without the mushrooms and then open freeze on a baking tray before placing in a container with greaseproof paper to separate. Defrost then warm through in the oven with fresh mushrooms, or sandwich in mini burger buns or stuff into pitta bread.

Experiment with the spicing for these – a little chipotle paste (1 teaspoon is around 8 cals) in place of the jalapeño would give a smokier taste, while adding a teaspoon each of ground cumin and ras al hanout (a Middle Eastern spice blend) would give a Moroccan twist.

CHAPTER EIGHT

Sides and sweets

The concept of 'snacking' isn't one I really endorse (see page 304 on meal timing) but sometimes you do need a low-calorie option to serve as a side dish, a sweet, or an emergency ration for if you get really hungry and want something that won't wreck your Fast Day. Everything in this chapter is easy, delicious and tasty – and all under 100 calories.

RECIPES

SMACKED CUCUMBER SALAD WITH GARLIC AND CHILLI,
🍺🥕🌾, 35

SESAME SEA VEGETABLE SALAD, 🍺🥕🌾, 92

NOOCH SPICED POPCORN, 🍺🥕🌾, 86

PURPLE CHILLI KIMCHI-KRAUT, 🍺🥕🌾, 25

ROAST SPICED CHICKPEAS, 🍺🥕🌾, 61

EDAMAME, ORANGE AND GINGER POT, 🍺🥕🌾, 90

AVOCADO CHOCBERRY MOUSSE, 🍺🥕🌾, 91

STRAWBERRY AND WATERMELON MARGARITA SALAD,
🍺🥕🌾, 68

RASPBERRY BAKEWELL ICE CREAM, 🍺🥕🌾, 56

GRIDDLED ALMOND NECTARINE, 🍺🥕🌾, 93

TROPICAL FRUIT CARPACCIO WITH COCONUT
AND GINGER CREAM, 🍺🥕🌾, 54

5:2 Lives

HEIKE'S THE BOSS OF HER BODY
AND 5 STONE (33KG) DOWN!

This is much more than I was hoping for. I love my body for going with me on this journey.'

Before: too big for sport or to play with her kids
After: fitter, lighter, able to go to the play park and join in

Heike hated her weight, and all the things it stopped her doing – especially with her three children. At the age of just 33, she was obese, and getting bigger.

'Before 5:2, I felt like a Buddha. At my heaviest, I weighed nearly 19 stone 9lb (125kg). I couldn't take my kids, who were then nine, four and two, to the indoor playground because I was too big to fit through the obstacles. Yet no one knew how to help me, not even my doctor, who is a long-term friend of mine.'

Because of the risk to her joints, Heike couldn't jog or try exercise. She felt stuck, and afraid. Then a friend tried 5:2 and suggested Heike did the same.

'She had lost weight... and felt invincible. So, one evening, she called me and said she knew how to help me to get rid of enough weight to start sports again. I thought, could it be that easy?'

Heike decided to go for it, and her first Fast Day did indeed turn out to be easy. 'I didn't expect that I'd be able to do it so I went into it feeling relaxed. I was working a 10-hour day in my job as a master optician, so I simply didn't take food to work, occupied myself with reading Kate's 5:2 book, and bought zucchini, mushrooms and chicken breast for dinner.'

Though Heike isn't completely vegetarian, she's switched to eating vegetarian food on Fast Days, and eats a lot less meat on non-fasting days, too. 'Being veggie makes me feel better and it's so much easier to fill my plate with vegetarian foods on Fast Days.'

So far, Heike has lost 5 stone (33kg) and she's down to 14 stone 6lb (92kg), which means she can exercise again. She can also buy normal clothes in the shops. But the health results have been the most dramatic. 'I can live my life more easily… I have no more blood pressure problems, no medicines for anything. No gout, my joints ache less, and hopefully I won't need new knees in ten years, as I would have before.

'I can carry the youngest, and the shopping, I do not snore, I sleep deeper and wake up more regenerated. And of course, now I can go to the indoor playground with the children.'

Heike, who lives in Lichtenstein, Germany, also encouraged her mother to try fasting. 'She's lost 2 stone 5lb (15kg) in half a year. No counting, no strict Fast Day routine. If she feels like having one on the same day as me, she asks me to prepare more food in the evening and we eat together.'

Heike wants to be back to around 11 stone 11lb (75kg), the weight she was at 18. 'I will never be a gazelle, but my husband Marco loves curves. This is much more than I was hoping for. I love my body for going with me on this journey.'

Fast Day routine:

I have to get up at 5.30. With a coffee, it is easier to get started! Then I keep myself busy. If you're too close to the fridge and your hands aren't busy, a very bad idea. When starting 5:2 I started counting calories. It made me mad, realising that such a small kid's yogurt had so much sugar and cals... So the content of our fridge is changing, too, slowly but steadily. For lunch, I eat nothing: I consume a good book instead, or have a good talk, drink a tea, write an email. I am usually at home at 20.30. The kids are normally in bed, so it's a goodnight kiss, then cooking my meals. I love to have a large plate, so I eat lots of veggies: zucchini, egg, mushrooms, cauliflower, tomatoes, spinach, stem cabbage, fennel, then natural low-fat yogurt with frozen fruits.

The other 5 days:

I'm more adventurous in testing new food. More veggies which I never tried. I do still eat things like noodles, mozzarella cheese, Greek yogurt, and of course chocolate, ice cream and Nutella... But I don't have the same appetite any more. Though after growing up in the GDR (East Germany), throwing away food makes me mad, which means psychologically I feel compelled sometimes to empty my plate. I am doing my best to change and to stop eating when I feel full.

The veggie life:

When I visited my veggie friend in June, I realised I eat 80 per cent veggie already. I am quite new to this way of eating and I'm not a hardliner: my main reason was a fuller plate and the delicious taste: it's so good, my children ask for Fast Day food on Non Fast Days.

Top tips:

Stick to the Fast Day calories limit, and to the two Fast Days for 8 weeks before going back to scale or measuring. Don't give up. Just change one thing at a time.

Last word:

I feel so much more self-confident. Eating is nice, fun and delicious. But it won't solve problems. Now I am the boss of my body.

SMACKED CUCUMBER SALAD WITH GARLIC AND CHILLI, 35 calories

I've been on the fence about cucumber for years, and then I tasted this, in the home of a Chinese friend, and it all made sense. 'Smacking' the cucumber – literally bashing it with a rolling pin! – breaks up the flesh and allows the simple, very spicy marinade to sink in. A medium cucumber makes 2 portions, and you can keep one, covered, in the fridge for 24 hours.

Serves 2
Preparation time: 5 minutes
Marinating time: 60+ minutes

    1 cucumber, around 250g, 35
    1 tablespoon rice vinegar, 3
    1 small garlic clove, chopped, 3
    ½ teaspoon salt, 0
    ½ teaspoon sugar, 8
    1 teaspoon soy or tamari sauce, 3–10
    ½ red chilli, finely chopped, 2–4, or 1 teaspoon chilli powder
        or flakes, 5
    3g lightly crushed peanuts, 17, to garnish

1. Lightly strike the cucumber with a rolling pin then with your hands pull it apart, break it into small chunks and place them in a bowl.

2. Mix the remaining ingredients in a jam jar with a lid, give the dressing a good shake, then pour over cucumber, mixing well to ensure it's coated. Leave to marinate at room temperature for up to 1 hour, then refrigerate until needed.

3. Sprinkle the nuts over the top to serve.

P. S. Serve as a side dish to accompany any of the Chinese and Korean dishes.

SESAME SEA VEGETABLE SALAD, 92 calories

Sea vegetables are a tiny bit magical, transforming from a few delicate leaves into a bowl full of multi-coloured seaweed in minutes and with barely any effort. Our neighbour's daughter Mackenzie brought this recipe back from a trip to Tokyo: the sesame dressing is the perfect accompaniment to the marine flavour of the veg. But I know sea veg aren't to everyone's taste, so try a small pack before filling the larder. You can buy them in Asian groceries, health food shops and online, such as from Amazon.

Serves 1
Preparation time: 10 minutes

¼ packet (around 10g) dried sea vegetables of your choice, around 20

For the dressing

1 teaspoon sesame oil, 41
1½ teaspoons soy or tamari sauce, 5–13
1½ teaspoons rice vinegar, 1
2cm/5g piece fresh ginger, peeled and grated, 4
1–2 drops agave syrup or a pinch of sugar, to taste, 3
Sea salt, to taste
1 small spring onion, chopped, to garnish, 2
½ teaspoon sesame seeds, 16 to garnish

1. Rinse the sea vegetables well, then rehydrate in a bowl using lukewarm water.

2. Meanwhile, make the dressing by combining the oil, soy or tamari, vinegar and ginger – taste to see if you need to add a little sweetness from the agave or sugar.

3. Squeeze out excess water from the sea vegetables and toss in the dressing, mixing well. Sprinkle the chopped spring onion and sesame seeds on the top.

P. S. There are so many different varieties of sea vegetable, so experiment until you find your favourite. Try adding chilli to the dressing for more of a kick.

NOOCH SPICED POPCORN, 86 calories

I've already raved about 'nooch' – nutritional yeast – and this is where it becomes the star of the show. For something good for you, nooch gives an almost fast-food flavour – think Cheesy Wotsits, but nicer. You can air-pop the corn, but without oil, the nooch won't stick – gently grinding the flakes also helps. You'll need an airtight container for this, to help coat the corn.

Serves 2, 86 per serving
Preparation time: 1 minute
Cooking time: 4–5 minutes

> 1 teaspoon butter, 36, or coconut or rapeseed/groundnut oil, 41
> 30g unpopped corn kernels or maize, 118
> 4 teaspoons nutritional yeast, around 4g, 14
> ¼ teaspoon cayenne pepper or ½ teaspoon turmeric, 3
> *Optional: finely ground sea salt, to taste*

1. Heat a medium saucepan with a lid and melt the butter or oil.

2. Pour the corn kernels or maize into the pan and shake so the oil coats them. Put the lid on and heat: after 1–3 minutes the corn will begin to pop. Shake a little as it does and wait at least 1 minute until it's stopped popping.

3. Meanwhile, mix together the nooch and spice in a pestle and mortar, and grind until the flakes turn into a powder.

4. Place half the flavour mix in a large plastic container, add the warm corn, sprinkle over the remaining nooch or spice, and replace the lid. Shake gently to distribute the flavouring: the oil and the moisture will help the nooch to stick. Eat immediately or store in the container for up to a week: any longer and it can go soggy.

P. S. Try other spices mixed with the nooch: ground cumin or ras al hanout are both warm and spicy.

PURPLE CHILLI KIMCHI-KRAUT, 25 calories

Fermented foods are all the rage – they're tangy, tasty and help to reintroduce 'friendly' bacteria into the gut. This recipe is a combination of sauerkraut and Korean kimchi, and has a glorious purple colour and a spicy kick. It's great with any dish as a relish or salad. You can buy gochugaru flakes online or at Asian groceries.

You'll need a plastic food bag for the very de-stressing process of pounding and crushing the veg by hand, plus glass jar (s) for the pickle: I used a 1-litre Kilner jar.

If you're new to fermented foods, eat small portions at first. They can be quite potent!

Makes 10 servings, 25 per serving
Preparation time: 15 minutes
Fermentation time: 7+ days

1 red cabbage, around 750g, shredded, 195
1 large/2 small carrots, around 100g, finely sliced into
    matchsticks, 34
2 garlic cloves, 8
1 tablespoon sea salt
1 tablespoon chilli powder or gochugaru Korean chilli flakes, 15

1. Wash the jars in hot soapy water to sterilise them, then put them in an oven heated to 140°C/275°F/Gas mark 1 until completely dry (remove the rubber seals before putting them in the oven or they'll melt).

2. In a large bowl, layer the veg, garlic, salt and chilli. Place your hand into the plastic food bag, to act as a glove, and use your hand to mix everything together really well – squash the vegetables into your fist, so that they begin to release their juices. Do this for 5–10 minutes then leave the veg to rest. Repeat after an hour or so, as many times as you like.

3. Pack the vegetables and their juices into the jars, pushing down thoroughly so there are no air pockets and the top of the veg is under the briny water the vegetables produced.

4. Allow to ferment at room temperature and open the jars every day or so to let gases escape. It's usually ready within 7 days, though fermentation time varies depending how warm the temperature is. The flavour will intensify over time but once it reaches your preferred strength, you can refrigerate the jars to slow the fermentation process.

NB: Always keep the veg submerged under the brine or it will go bad and spoil the whole batch: you can top up with water and a little more salt if the 'massaging' hasn't produced enough brine to cover.

P. S. This is also great served on top of oatcakes or slices of cucumber. Once you've tried the basic recipe, you can experiment with white or Chinese cabbage, add radishes, celeriac and other root vegetables, or add other flavours, such as fresh ginger, fresh chillies and spring onion.

ROAST SPICED CHICKPEAS, 61 calories

Chickpeas are so versatile, and these crunchy pulses make a fab pre-dinner or emergency snack for Fast Days – they also work well as a salad topping. They are also so quick and easy to prepare as the recipe uses tinned pulses.

Serves 6 as a snack, 61 per portion
Preparation time: 3 minutes
Cooking time: 30–35 minutes

1 x 400g tin chickpeas, drained, 312
1 teaspoon rapeseed/groundnut or coconut oil, 41
2 teaspoons ras al hanout spice mix or smoked paprika, 10
Sea salt, to taste

1. Preheat the oven to 200°C/400°F/Gas mark 6. Dry the drained chickpeas well on kitchen roll and give them a rub – it improves the texture if you remove any of the loose skins from the pulses. It's easy to remove them with your fingers, too, but don't worry if you don't have time or can't be bothered!

2. Take a non-stick roasting tin and pour in the oil. Tip the chickpeas into the tin and roll them around so they all get a light coating. Now sprinkle over the spices and roll around a second time. Season with salt.

3. Bake in the oven for 30 minutes and then check them – you want them dried out and crunchy but they can burn suddenly so make sure you keep a close eye towards the end of the cooking time. Remove them and serve

warm, or keep in an airtight container. They will soften a little but still taste good for up to 3 days.

P. S. The spice options are almost unlimited. For a simple salad, use these to top baby spinach leaves, adding a few sun-dried tomatoes (drain off the oil with kitchen roll), with a little tahini poured over.

EDAMAME, ORANGE AND GINGER POT, 90 calories

Simple but deeply flavoured, this pot of emerald-green beans with a sweet and savoury sesame dressing is great eaten either freshly cooked or at room temperature. It makes a good side or you can double the portion size for a very light lunch served with some bitter leaves, such as rocket or radicchio, and the flesh from the other half of the orange, cubed.

Serves 1
Preparation time: 10 minutes
Cooking time: 5 minutes

> 30g frozen edamame beans, 39
> 60g trimmed green beans, 19
> Juice and zest of ½ small orange, around 40ml, 15
> 1cm piece fresh ginger, peeled and grated, 2
> A sprinkling of sesame seeds, 5
> A few drops/¼ teaspoon sesame oil, 10
> Freshly ground sea salt and black pepper, to taste

1. Blanch the edamame and green beans in a pan of boiling water for 2 minutes. Drain, then plunge them into a bowl of cold water to stop further cooking. If you wish, pop the edamame out of their skins by squeezing them gently between finger and thumb.

2. Heat the orange juice and grated ginger in a small pan until simmering, then add the green vegetables and cook until the juice is slightly reduced. Pour onto a plate, scatter over the zest and a few sesame seeds plus the

sesame oil. Season, then serve immediately or at room temperature as a salad.

P. S. Use fine asparagus in place of the green beans for a 'posher' pot!

AVOCADO CHOCBERRY MOUSSE, 91 calories

(🍴) (🥕) (🌾) if agave nectar used

This has an intense dark chocolate flavour, plus the richness of avocado, and bright jewels of berry fruit mixed through. I've allowed for a little agave or honey to sweeten but if your berries are really sweet, you can leave that out. The cocoa powder prevents the avocado discolouring, but it's still best to eat these within a day of making. Keep them in the fridge, covered.

Serves 2
Preparation time: 4 minutes

- 40g sweet raspberries, blackberries, or both, defrosted if frozen, 21
- ½ large avocado or 1 small, very ripe, flesh weighing around 75g, 140
- ½–1 teaspoon (2–4g) cocoa powder or raw cacao powder, 5–10
- 1 teaspoon agave nectar or honey, 16–20, to sweeten

1. Reserve 2 berries for garnish and add the rest to a bowl with the avocado flesh and half the cocoa. Whip together, lightly crushing the berries – younger avocados may need to be mashed more forcefully!

2. Taste the mix and add more cocoa for a deeper chocolate flavour, or agave or honey for sweetness.

3. Spoon into small pots or espresso cups and top with the reserved berries. Refrigerate until you want to eat them.

P. S. This works well with blueberries, too, or for a different flavour, try with a quarter of a small orange (around 20 calories), finely chopped. You can also use the mousse as a delicious chocolatey spread on toast the next day!

STRAWBERRY AND WATERMELON MARGARITA SALAD, 68 calories

This really is more than the sum of its parts – a fruit salad, taking the flavours from Mexico's famous margarita cocktail, but instead of tequila, I've used agave nectar, produced from the same plant as tequila. If you don't have agave, use honey, though this means the dish won't be suitable for vegans. *So* refreshing.

Serves 1
Preparation time: 5 minutes plus 1+ hour refrigeration

Juice and zest of ½ lime, 8
½ teaspoon agave nectar, 7
75g strawberries, cut in half if large, 24
120g wedge watermelon (90g without rind), cut into cubes, 27
Optional garnish: a few tiny mint or basil leaves, 2

1. Mix the lime juice and agave in a bowl (save the squeezed lime half), add the fruits and mix gently to coat. Refrigerate for 1–5 hours (any longer and the fruit will become mushy).

2. Just before serving, grate the lime zest over the fruit and sprinkle with the herbs, if using.

P. S. This is also delicious with other melons or mango chunks (60 calories per 100g). On non-Fast Day, use a teaspoon of real tequila in the marinade…

RASPBERRY BAKEWELL ICE CREAM, 56 calories

These are wonderfully indulgent-tasting, but in reality they're low-calorie, super-quick and a good mini Fast Day dessert if you feel like one: you'll need either a robust hand blender, or a food processor. A great way to use up old bananas, too!

Makes 6
Preparation time: 5 minutes

> 3 small/2 large ripe bananas, around 275g, peeled, 289
> 85g fresh or frozen raspberries, 44
> ½ teaspoon almond extract, 1–5 depending on brand
> Also: 6 espresso cups, egg cups or rinsed fromage frais mini
>   pots

1. Peel the bananas then slice into chunks and freeze for 1–2 hours. If they've been frozen for a lot longer, let the chunks sit at room temperature for ten minutes to avoid damaging the processor or blender.

2. Reserve 6 whole raspberries, and process the rest of the raspberries first in the processor or blender beaker. Now add the almond extract and a third of the banana chunks and process/blend, followed by the other chunks as the mixture forms a smooth ice cream mix. If the blender is struggling, let the bananas thaw a little more or add a splash of almond or dairy milk.

3. Pour into pots and add a whole frozen raspberry to the centre of each.

4. You can either eat these now, or return them to the freezer for 10 minutes to freeze a little more.

5. Keep these in the freezer for up to 1 month: if not eating on the same day, seal the top with cling film and store the pots in a plastic box or sealed bag so they don't absorb other smells. If they have been frozen for some time, let them thaw for 10 minutes before serving.

P. S. To make a key lime and walnut version (65 per pot), replace the raspberries with 2 limes (30), 10g walnut pieces (65) and ½ teaspoon ground ginger (3). Zest and juice the limes and reserve 6 small pieces of walnut. Add the rest of the nuts to a food processor with the frozen banana pieces, lime juice and zest and the ground ginger and process as before, topping each pot with a walnut piece.

GRIDDLED ALMOND NECTARINE, 93 calories

Griddling or roasting fruit always intensifies the sweetness, and this simple dessert feels indulgent but fresh – it's also a good way of using underripe fruit that's slightly too firm to eat as it is. Nectarines are high in soluble fibre and such a stunning colour, too. If you don't have/like nectarines, you could use a peach instead.

Serves 1
Preparation time: 2 minutes
Cooking time: 2–3 minutes

A few drops of mild-flavoured oil, for greasing, 10
1 nectarine, not too ripe, halved and stone removed, 51

To serve

A few drops of almond extract, 1–2
1 level dessertspoon/10g Greek yogurt, 10,
    or coconut yogurt, 17
3 whole almonds, 21

1. Use kitchen roll to grease a small area of a griddle pan with the scantest amount of oil, then heat to a very high temperature.

2. Place the nectarine, cut side down, onto the hot pan. Cook for 2–3 minutes, until the fruit starts to caramelise – turn down the heat if it seems to be burning. Don't move the fruit, you want to get nice char marks from the griddle.

3. To serve, place the nectarine halves, cut side up, on a plate, drizzle over the almond extract and top with yogurt and nuts. Serve warm.

P. S. For a tropical variation, use coconut oil and replace the almonds with the flesh and seeds from a passion fruit (17) and a sprinkling of flaked toasted coconut, about 3g (18). On a non-Fast Day, serve with vanilla dairy/vegan ice cream and a crumbled amaretti biscuit. If you want to serve more than 1 person, roast the fruit in an ovenproof dish in an oven heated to 180°C/350°F/Gas mark 4 for 15 minutes, with the oil brushed on top.

TROPICAL FRUIT CARPACCIO WITH COCONUT AND GINGER CREAM, 54 calories

This is a tropical fruit salad made Fast Day-friendly. It works either as a very light lunch – increase the coconut yogurt to make it more filling – or a dessert. You can use one, two or three types of fruit (whatever's ripe or going cheap at the market) or a prepacked fruit multi-pack makes it doable for one person. You can wrap the leftover passion fruit half in cling film and use it the next day.

Serves 1, calories 54–120 depending on calories in fruit or yogurt
Preparation time: 5 minutes

> 100g fresh fruit, pineapple, mango, melon, starfruit, kiwi, strawberries, 30–60 (calories vary from 34 for honeydew melon, 50 for pineapple, 60 for mango)
> 25g coconut yogurt, 14–49
> Seeds from ½ passion fruit, 9
> Sprinkling of ground ginger, or a little peeled and grated fresh ginger, 1–2

1. Peel the fruit, if needed (i.e. pineapple, mango, kiwi). Using your sharpest knife, slice the fruits into the thinnest slices you can – we're aiming for thinner than packaged cheese slices.

2. Arrange the fruit in a circle on a plate, leaving a gap in the centre, then place the yogurt in the middle. Cut open the passion fruit and spread the seeds across the fruit and yogurt. Sprinkle or grate over the ginger.

P. S. Replace the yogurt with half a ball of reduced-fat mozzarella (100–109) or 15g mixed nuts (around 100) to make more a substantial salad dish. Low-fat plain cottage cheese, 18 per 25g, is also a nutritious option.

3

5:2
EATING WELL
FOR LIFE

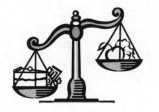

Fast Day
Meal Plans

The meal plans here are based on eating **two meals a day, plus a side dish that you could either eat as a separate light meal or at the same time as one of the other two meals.** The 'two meals' structure has consistently been the most popular option for members of our 50,000-strong 5:2 Facebook group. Of course, you're free to choose your own meal timings, using the guidance on page 304. The real-life stories from 5:2 veggies in each recipe chapter also show how it works in practice.

The total calorie consumptions per day are based on around 500 calories per day, which is the recommendation for women.

Extra options for men:

Men can have around 100 calories extra per day, taking their allowance to 600. Choose your own options from the following, or look at the recipes for inspiration – especially those under 100 calories (see page 340). Avoid eating snacks or ready-made cakes or diet foods.

Meal extras		Fruit and veg	
Poached or boiled egg	66	100g cooked spinach	25
Veggie sausage	70–100	100g cooked broccoli	32
80g tofu	92+	½ vacuum pack beetroot	53
10g nuts or seeds	56–70	½ very small avocado, 50g flesh	80
25g full-fat cheese	60–100	100g chestnut mushrooms fried in ½ teaspoon butter	40
25g lower-fat cheese (e.g. ricotta, light feta)	34–70	100g cherry tomatoes and 10g rocket with 1 tablespoon balsamic vinegar	30–40
50g full-fat Greek yogurt	48–65	50g raspberries	26
Very thin slice of bread (weigh), 25g	55–63	1 kiwi fruit	42
Small portion (25g uncooked) grains, e.g. rice, barley, farro	86–95	1 small banana	89–100

Seasonal menus

SPRING

Spicy flavoured feast: (🌾), 489

Lunch: Vietnamese spicy pho with fresh herbs and courgette
noodles, 70
Supper: Gado gado Indonesian egg salad with hot peanut
sauce, 252
Meal 3/starter/side: Smacked cucumber salad with garlic and
chilli, 35, Edamame, orange and ginger pot, 90, small kiwi
fruit, 42

Italian flavour: (🌾), 508
Lunch: 2 rocket and ricotta frittata muffins, 158, with 20g baby
spinach, 50g tomatoes, 1 tablespoon balsamic vinegar, 20
Dinner: Courgetti carbonara with asparagus, 247
Meal 3/starter/side: Fragrant tomato broth with fresh herbs, 97

5 a day: (🥜) (🌾), 475
Lunch: Fresh corn and black bean tacos, 247
Supper: Hot aubergine and pepper perfect stir-fry, 155
Meal 3/starter/side: Broccoli soup, 73

Stateside brunch and salad day: (🥚), 502
Brunch: Homemade baked beans on toast, 195
Supper: Veggie version of Rainbow Cobb salad, 271
Meal 3/starter/side: 75g mushrooms sautéed in ½ teaspoon
butter or oil, 35–40

SUMMER

Summer's best: ⬭, 496

Lunch: Carrot and lemon hummus salad jar, 140, with
portion of kimkraut, 38
Supper: Individual tomato and onion tarte tatin and rocket
salad, 225
Meal 3/starter/side: Griddled almond nectarine, 93

Indian Fast Day: ⬭⬭, 508
Lunch: Onion bhaji lunchbox omelette, 179
Supper: Paneer tikka masala, 301
Meal 3/starter/side: cauli rice cooked with fresh coriander
and chilli flakes, 28

Cheese, please: ⬭, 510
Lunch: Halloumi salad with melon, cucumber and mint, 203
Supper: Warm beluga lentils with homemade yogurt cheese,
255
Meal 3/starter/side: pop-art coleslaw, 52

Salad days: ⬭⬭, 487
Lunch: Sweet and sour aubergine caponata with pear, 131,
with head of Little Gem lettuce, 15
Supper: Black rice salad with beetroot, orange and kefir, 287
Meal 3/starter/side: Tropical fruit carpaccio with coconut
and ginger cream, 54

AUTUMN

Autumn harvest: (icon),486

Lunch: Herby wild mushroom parcels on toast, 155
Supper: Rich aubergine parmigiana, 273
Meal 3/starter/side: artichoke pâté with grilled red chicory, 58

A celebration of herbs and spices: (icon), 501
Lunch: Hiker's hearty bean and leek soup with hot paprika, 121
Supper: Roasted field mushrooms with farro wheat and kale, 249
Meal 3/starter/side: Mini beetroot sliders with slaw, 131

Avocado delights: (icon), 491
Lunch: Stuffed avocado, 209
Supper: Open butternut squash lasagne with almond vegan pesto, 191
Meal 3/starter/side: avocado chocberry mousse, 91

Sharing weekend: (icon)(icon)(icon), 506
Lunch: Kale and paprika falafel with pomegranate and harissa drizzle, 152
Supper: Roasted cauliflower steak Italian-style, 179, and butternut mash, 40
Meal 3/starter/side: Carrot hummus, 92; 1 oatcake crackers, 43

WINTER

Winter warmers: (icon), 406

Lunch: Senegalese spicy squash and peanut stew, 220
Supper: Yorkshire puds with sage and mustard mushrooms, 211
Meal 3/starter/side: Coconut spinach, 35, 1 small tangerine, 40

Spiceworld: (icon)(icon), 481

Lunch: Peacamole mint tostadas with red pepper, 218
Supper: Thai Jungle curry with baby corn and tofu, 238
Meal 3/starter/side: Cauli rice, 25

Chilli peppers, (icon)(icon), 502

Lunch: Puy lentil stuffed Ramiro peppers, 258
Supper: sweet potato chilli, 224
Meal 3/starter/side: 50g blackberries, 20

East Asian savouries: (icon)(icon) option, 517

Lunch: Super-savoury miso aubergine, 163
Supper: noodles, 263
Meal 3/starter/side: Sesame sea vegetable salad, 92

2-meal/2-course meal Fast Day ideas

For days when you want a two-course meal, perhaps when eating with friends or family, these work a treat.

Warming dinner menu: ⊘, 509
Starter/light meal: chickpea and wild mushroom warmer soup, 142, thin 25g slice bread, 56
Main meal: Jerk tofu steaks, 276, and coconut spinach, 35

Chinese takeaway (pick either starter or dessert): ⊘, 465
Starter/light meal: Mushroom and mangetout soup with miso noodles, 146
Main meal: Chinese pancakes, 247
Dessert: 1 kiwi fruit (aka the Chinese gooseberry), 42, with 10g goji berries, 30

Trip to Latin America (pick either starter or dessert): ⊛, 469
Starter/light dish: Smoked chilli velvet soup (version made with sweet potato), 126
Main meal: Mushroom and yellow chilli quinotto risotto with white wine, ⊕⊘⊛, 275
Dessert: Strawberry and watermelon margarita salad, 68

Indian big brunch: ⊛, 487
Brunch: 1 Indian chilli breakfast pancake, 120, dal, 280, 1 egg fried in ½ teaspoon coconut oil, 87.

Family and friends weekend: (icons), **470**
Brunch: Pea and herb pancakes with watercress and poached eggs, 222
Dinner: Squash and sage roast, 224, 75g steamed broccoli, 24

Vegan BBQ: (icons), **490**
1 Chestnut, leek and mushroom 'sausage' roll, 144
1 portion mini beetroot sliders with slaw, 131
BBQ Kumara and beets with a creamy pistachio dukkah topping, 215

Vegan fast-food weekend: (icons), **501–533**
Beany Bunn, aka curry sandwich, 268
Gluten-free crispy socca pizza, 193, with your choice of vegan
   toppings, 40–72

The other five days: how to make non-Fast Days work for you

Fast Days give your body and mind a break from overload, but what about non-fasting days? Should we just carry on eating as before – or take steps to eat better on the five days, too?

A balanced diet

On your non-fasting days, ideally, you'll eat a balanced diet with plenty of vegetables, wholegrains and healthy fats. But that doesn't mean you'll always be eating a 'perfect' diet – your days vary: sometimes you might be too busy to eat much, or just not feel hungry. On others – especially celebrations or on holiday – you might include some less healthy but still delicious foods, or drink alcohol.

Most people find when they do 5:2 they become more conscious of what they're eating on the other 5 days, so they are less likely to snack without thinking, and are also more aware of portion size and calories. I remember once seeing a cake that was over 500 calories – more than I'd eaten in total the previous day. It just didn't seem worth it.

On non-fasting days, I've never calorie-counted every meal. But I do keep in mind an overall idea of what my body needs (and I know my TDEE, see page 47) and aim to balance out the days when I have too much, say at a party or during a weekend away, with non-fasting days where I'm a bit more careful. This is sustainable for me, and less boring than counting the whole time.

But what if your idea of what's 'enough' has become completely distorted?

Portion distortion: re-educating yourself about what your body needs

The reasons behind weight gain are complex, but for most of us, the bottom line is we were eating more than our bodies needed, and we stored the excess as fat. The calorie gap from Fast Days will help, but if you've been overeating for years – or even decades – you will need some guidance on what's appropriate for you.

Your TDEE as a guideline

This is where your TDEE comes in (see page 47 for how to calculate it). It isn't an exact science, but if you've been eating excessively for a long time it will help you check what the right amount of food is for your size, activity levels and lifestyle.

I still wouldn't suggest calorie-counting every day. Instead, keep a food diary for a few days – including weekdays and weekend days, as eating patterns tend to be different day to day – and tot up the calories in that. Weigh your food rather than estimate it and then compare that to your TDEE. If you're way over, look at:

- **Portion size** – is it easier to reduce this, rather than make something else you don't like?
- **Cooking and preparation methods** – can you cut down on the fat you're using with bread or when cooking? Can you apply some of the Fast Day ideas from page 293?
- **Sugary and processed foods** – you don't need to cut out all sweet things and takeaways, but could they be an occasional part of your diet rather than featuring on most days?
- Are you including a bare **minimum of 5 portions of vegetables, beans or pulses and fruit** per day? Look for opportunities to replace some higher-calorie foods with fresh produce: could you replace chips with carrots, crisps with crudités?

Above all, don't ban any foods; try to set positive goals, not negative rules. I enjoy chocolate, cheese, treats, celebratory meals and wine, and I've lost 20 per cent of my body weight, *and* maintained that loss.

Metabolism matters

Earlier in the book, we explored how short-term fasting can speed up metabolism; metabolism influences how fast we lose weight, and whether we regain it.

Metabolism basics

Metabolism describes all the chemical processes in the body that keep us alive, including growing, renewing cells and using energy. In the media, it's often used to mean *just* the process of breaking down the food we eat to give us energy. That energy is then used in our daily activities, to help us repair or renew our cells and systems, or it can be stored as glycogen (for rapid fuel) or fat. Our TDEE is calculated by looking at the factors that influence metabolism, including our weight, age, sex and activity levels.

Metabolism facts and myths

- There are two ways to speed up your metabolism: becoming more muscular, or raising the heartbeat.
- Eating more regularly has not been proven to raise the metabolism (despite the common advice that we should eat mini meals all the time).
- Short-term fasting may raise metabolism temporarily in some people as adrenalin, and therefore heart rate, can increase in the first couple of days. We don't yet know if this happens every time you fast, or whether the body becomes accustomed to it: it may vary from person to person.

What about starvation mode? And yo-yo dieting?

'Starvation mode' is talked about a lot by dieters – the fear is that by lowering their calorie intake for one or two days their body will 'hoard' energy and undo all their good work. But the truth is, your body is highly unlikely to do this because you're mixing up the fasts with days when you're not restricting.

Over time, as you lose weight, your Basal Metabolic Rate *does* reduce a little, because there's actually less of you to carry around, which takes less energy.

What does seem increasingly important is trying to keep as close to your ideal weight as possible, as yo-yo dieting – going up and down over time – can negatively affect your metabolism. If you've dieted several times to reach your goal weight, you may need fewer calories than someone who weighs the same but has always been the same size. This isn't specific to 5:2 or intermittent fasting, but it's another reason to try to find a weight-loss method that works for you, long-term.

Combining 5:2 with other diets to lose weight faster

In our Facebook group, people often ask if they can combine this tool or way of eating with other diet plans. Frequently those who've had success with 'standard 5:2' can be critical, because they're so pleased with how it's worked for them.

For me, it's not quite that simple. There are some commercial diets that offer very sensible guidelines on healthy eating, and can help us re-educate our palates and appetites, but personally, I am wary of meal replacements, as they're often high in sugar and don't retrain us to look for 'real' food.

I would suggest that if you do restrict calories on non-fasting days, don't set the calorie limit too low – this is mainly for reasons of sustainability, because you want to be able to stick to it and not feel deprived. For women, I'd suggest not going under 1200 calories on non-fasting days and for men, 1500.

Cutting out carbs – as diets like Atkins or South Beach do – can speed up weight loss, but it is hard to maintain, especially as a vegetarian, because so many plant-based meals and good grains contain carbs. It is possible, and I sometimes reduce the amount of bread, rice and other grains, and replace them with more green veggies just before a holiday or special occasion, but it can be unbalanced long-term, so it's better used as a short-term strategy. Cutting out an entire food group is not the answer for most of us.

Time-restricted approaches to eating

You might have heard of 16:8 alongside 5:2 – it's where you're advised to eat only in an 8-hour window per day, say from 11am to 7pm. It's one version of time-restricted eating – limiting the times when we allow ourselves to eat, and might be a natural partner for intermittent fasting. Intermittent fasting pioneer Dr Krista Varady was part of a team that reviewed studies of what they called 'time-restricted feeding'; for example, only eating during a 'window' that might last between three to twelve hours. They concluded that there may be benefits in terms of reduced body weight *and* improved results in health tests.

There could be different reasons for this:

- You have fewer chances to overdo it/overeat.
- The pancreas will be secreting less insulin, allowing you to burn stored fat.
- The shorter periods of eating/digesting food may create mini-fasts that encourage healing and repair.

Meal timing/frequency tips

- **Avoid snacking and eating between meals** unless advised otherwise by a medical professional (see below).
- **Work out what suits you best,** if you **love breakfast** and find it stops you eating processed or higher-calorie foods later, stick with it. But if you **don't enjoy eating first thing** and feel more able to eat nutritious meals by delaying eating until later, follow your appetite.
- **Consider** incorporating longer gaps between meals, like the 16:8 approach outlined above. This creates some 'mini-fasts' where your body isn't constantly digesting food/using insulin to control blood sugar. There may be a metabolic advantage – speeding up our body's processes – and it might also aid the cellular 'housekeeping' I've talked about elsewhere. But do be aware that it's still possible to consume plenty of calories/energy in 8 hours, so as a weight-LOSS strategy, it may not always work.
- **Whatever time of day you're eating, focus on making good food choices;** aim for fresh produce with minimal processing or additives.

If I had one single piece of advice on controlling appetite and eating better, it would be the first point: **reduce or cut out snacks entirely**, unless you've been advised differently by your GP or medical team – for instance, this might be the case if you have insulin-dependent diabetes or are on frequent medication that can't be taken on an empty stomach.

Positive about food: achieving balance on non-fasting days

Of course, calories aren't the whole story. Even a wholly veggie or vegan diet can be unhealthy – I've known veggies who exist on toast, chips, takeaway veggie burgers and ice cream. Even though they *might* not be eating enough to put on weight, it was never going to deliver on nutrition.

You'll find some sample menus below (based on what I eat on a non-fasting day) to give you an idea of non-fasting days in practice. My regime now is to fast once a week – usually on a Monday – but to increase to two a week after a holiday, or if I feel my clothes becoming a little tighter…

Kate's non-fasting day menus

A typical non-fasting week day in winter

Breakfast/brunch (if I have a busy day ahead): Small bowl of full-fat Greek yogurt with fresh or frozen berries or compote, such as blackberries and blueberries, topped with ground flaxseed and walnut mix.

OR

2 slices wholemeal sourdough bread with butter and peanut butter or half an avocado.

Lunch: Bowl of homemade veggie soup with a topping, such as crème fraiche, grated cheese, toasted seeds or served with a slice of sourdough.

OR

An omelette/Spanish omelette slice with side salad, dressed with olive oil and balsamic vinegar with some seeds.

Small handful of nuts (such as 6 walnuts or 6 almonds or 8 pistachios or 5 Brazils).

Small piece of fruit, such as kiwi, apple, pear.

Supper: A bowl of veggie curry with beans, tofu or paneer with a small serving of basmati rice or mixed with another grain, such as quinoa or farro, plus Greek yogurt and chutney, topped with coriander.

OR

A mushroom risotto or spicy tomato pasta dish, with more vegetables than grains, grated Grana Padano, served with a salad.

OR

Homemade cauli and broccoli cheese with garlic bread or tomato salad.

I also have 1 glass of red wine 1–2 nights. 1 small cake/vegan almond choc brownie/25g dark chocolate, 1–2 days a week after lunch or supper on the days I don't have wine.

A typical non-fasting weekend day (more indulgent) in winter

Brunch: Eggs Florentine at my favourite café – 2 poached eggs, 2 slices sourdough toast, freshly cooked spinach, hollandaise sauce made with butter and eggs, a few seeds on top.

Evening meal: Night out at local restaurant – perhaps some olives and pepper/artichoke antipasti, followed by a thin-crust pizza with vegetables and cheese, a side salad with extra-virgin olive oil dressing and a portion of ice-cream, with 2–3 glasses of red wine.

OR

a curry – bhel poori yogurt and chopped vegetable salad with puffed grains, then a dal, spinach paneer or vegetable korma with half a portion of rice, with 2 gin and slimline tonics.

A typical 16:8 day in winter

Often I eat two meals in a day, rather than three: it suits me well.

Brunch/lunchtime: Veggie full English with mushrooms, egg fried in butter, and either halloumi or avocado, seeds sprinkled on top.

Evening: veggie stir-fry in sesame oil with tofu and sriracha sauce, sesame seeds on top.

OR

Jacket sweet potato with a salad, mixed chilli beans and some crème fraiche.

A typical non-fasting weekday in summer

Breakfast: Greek yogurt and chopped strawberries and nectarine, topped with ground flaxseed and walnut mix.

OR

2 slices wholemeal sourdough bread with butter and peanut butter or half an avocado

Lunch: Homemade salad, such as avocado and mozzarella salad or homemade hummus with spring onions and sourdough bread or crackers, topped with seeds or nuts.

OR

Takeaway of four fresh salads from local veggie take-away, e.g. spiced carrot coleslaw, pak choi salad with sesame and soy, chickpea and spinach, rocket and tomato, topped with seeds and hummus.

Supper: Roasted pepper quiche with steamed broccoli or peas, and a few sweet potato wedges/oven chips or new potatoes with a knob of butter.

OR

Farro salad with summer vegetables: asparagus, artichoke antipasti, olive oil and lemon, plus toasted pine nuts.

OR

Black lentil salad with beetroot and goat's cheese topped with pecans or pistachios.

OR

Falafel, tahini, wholemeal pitta bread, salad dressed with pomegranate molasses and sesame seeds.

As in winter, I'll have wine 1–2 weeknights, or a small piece of chocolate or cake once or twice on the days I don't have wine.

A typical 16:8 day in summer

Brunch: Homemade or shop-made bircher muesli with apple, cinnamon and yogurt.

OR

Hot grilled avocado on toast with cherry tomatoes and sweet chilli sauce.

Evening: Griddled halloumi with grilled vegetables, olive oil, a grain side dish such as tabbouleh (bulgur wheat, tomato and herbs) or rice/quinoa salad with pomegranate seeds or oranges.

A typical non-fasting weekend day (more indulgent) in summer

Breakfast: At local café, such as Huevos Rancheros (Mexican eggs).

Evening: Nuts or crisps and a cocktail or glass of cava at home.

Dinner: at favourite pub or veggie restaurant with half bottle of wine, such as vegetable pho at Vietnamese restaurant, with spicy crackers.

OR

Beer-battered halloumi with fries and peas, and usually a starter, or possibly a dessert instead.

That's *my* version: enjoy the freedom to create your own 'normal'.

I'm not saying that any of this is perfect diet for you, but I want you to see what's realistic. I do drink wine up to three nights a week and I typically have chocolate or something sweet a couple of non-fasting days, too. On most 'full-time' diets, those would be seen as bad choices, even sinful. I see them as delicious, but not for every single day.

Some days I have more than two slices of toast... often the day before my period! My approach certainly isn't 'clean-eating' – a phrase I loathe – but it's good food, either made at home or from shops and restaurants I know and trust, with the occasional processed/frozen meal or soup for convenience.

The other thing to notice is it's not *that* different to what I'm suggesting you eat on a Fast Day – it's just a more generous portion, or I have bread or grains as a side, or I add a little more olive oil or some nutritious nuts or seeds to the dressing. And, of course, I don't have wine or sweet things on a Fast Day because that'd mean I couldn't eat the more nutritious dishes in this book!

Weight maintenance

Losing weight is sometimes easier than keeping it off – some studies suggest a third of people who lose weight on conventional diets will regain weight, while others say it's 80 per cent! And many people actually end up heavier than they were before they dieted, which can be utterly disheartening.

The reasons include:

- **Lower energy needs after dieting:** When we're lighter, we need fewer calories *unless* we become more active to balance that out. If we fail to realise this, we can easily put the weight back on.

- **Diet fatigue:** Many conventional dieters need to calorie-count full-time, even after their period 'on a diet' is over – it's tiresome and can feel like a life sentence. Plus, if you suddenly have the freedom to eat previously 'banned' foods, it's easy to go overboard and return to old habits.
- **Effects of dieting on metabolism and hunger/ appetite regulation:** Yo-yo dieting can affect the metabolism after a diet ends, though we don't know if it's permanent.

I always regained weight after diets – until 5:2. Now I stay within 2–3 pounds of my lowest 5:2 weight, even though I was recently diagnosed with an underactive thyroid which slows down the metabolism and can make people GAIN weight.

So why has 5:2 been different after decades of failure? Because the ease and health benefits of 5:2 have made me want to incorporate fasting into my routine for life. As I've explained, I still fast once every week – because it makes me feel great, has those same protective health effects, and gives me a reminder of all those signals our body sends but that we're sometimes too busy to hear.

Simple strategies for maintaining your weight loss

If you see fasting as a beneficial habit you'll want to use it as a tool to maintain a healthy weight permanently. There are different ways to achieve this:

- **6:1** Fasting one day each week is the most obvious

way to do it because it will help you stay aware of the benefits of fasting and how you can learn to trust your appetite. It will also help smooth over any days when you might overdo it, such as holidays or social events.

- **Flexi-fasting** This is what I do. I trust my instincts on how much I've eaten out and exercised the previous week, then I adjust my number of fasting days accordingly. Mostly I'll do one Fast Day, but if I've been overindulging, I switch to two until my clothes are looser. And I never fast on holiday!
- **Other scheduled eating approaches** such as 16:8 (see page 303). Since 5:2 has taken off, lots of other approaches have appeared that use time as a diet tool, such as limiting when you eat.

Monitoring your weight is also important – though it doesn't mean being a slave to the scales. You know yourself whether you'll be upset if your weight fluctuates if you weigh yourself. If the figures are a bit of a minefield for you, find a pair of jeans or dress that fits perfectly at your ideal weight and try it on if you feel you might be slipping – they'll tell you for sure.

If you're comfortable with weighing yourself, once or twice a week is about right, at the same time of day and ideally *on* the same day(s) too.

Fasting: A strategy, not a straitjacket

The important thing to remind yourself about 5:2 and intermittent fasting is that it should fit in around you; it's a strategy, not a straitjacket. You can use it to fit your life – if you're used to very strict diets this can be disorientating at first but it's what makes it sustainable and customisable for you. As you learn which frequency and pattern of fasting/normal eating works for you, you'll grow in confidence and understand why this approach has been adopted for life by so many people.

Mental tips for long-term success

Whether you're new to fasting, or it's a part of your life now, it's good to have a final reminder of how your attitude and focus can be the key to success.

Keep a record: Dieters who keep a record of what they eat tend to be more successful. You can either do that electronically, or jot it down in a notebook. An app/site like **myfitnesspal. com** makes it easy to record your consumption on Fast Days. You simply enter the name of the food (or scan barcodes on packaging) and the app calculates the calories. It'll also **keep track of weight loss over time.** There's no 5:2 setting, so the easiest option is to set your membership to Maintain, but limit yourself to 500/600 calories on Fast Days.

- Use your notes to **personalise your approach**: review which days, meal timings and dishes made you feel great, and which didn't work so well. Learning from your successes – and challenges – will keep things fresh.
- Control **your eating environment**. Sit down at the table to eat your meals rather than eating in front of the TV or while travelling.

- **Remind yourself about the health benefits of fasting** to motivate you. See page 12 or follow links to the studies in the resources section in Part 4.
- **Take advantage of the mental focus fasting can give**: Plan to do absorbing, interesting tasks on Fast Days – you may perform better than on normal days.
- **Don't give up...** there will be days I've dubbed T.I.T.S-U.P. Days (Temporary Interruption To Scheme, Un-Planned) when a planned fast goes wrong. You might get bad news, or even good, and decide not to continue the fast.
- The secret is to **take it a day at a time**: the occasional slip-up won't damage your health or your long-term success. **Just plan a new fast**, and take control again.
- **Focus on the future, not the past...**

Fastiversaries: something to celebrate

I have one final tip for making this a life change and not just a quick fix. Make a note of when you have your first fast – and then, each year, celebrate your *Fastiversary!* It's the name I've given to the anniversary of your first fast, but you should also give yourself a pat on the back at one, two, three or six months.

With every other diet, I've ever tried, the idea of *celebrating* being on it after a year or more would have seemed crazy. But the health and mindful-eating benefits of 5:2 mean every Fastiversary marks another year of doing something proactive for your health and future.

5:2 Lives

2 STONE LOST, 50,000 NEW FRIENDS
AND A VEGGIE DREAM COME TRUE

5:2 has changed my life in every single way.

Before: yo-yo dieter worried about a health and weight time-bomb
After: happier, lighter, free to enjoy my 5:2 life

Lifelong veggie Kate, from Brighton, had been on the weight-loss rollercoaster all her adult life when she tried fasting as a last-ditch attempt to get into better shape…

She… **hold on.**

OK, I admit it, this is *my* story. I've told it so many times since writing my first book about 5:2 in November 2012, but my publisher suggested it might be fun to bring things bang up to date!

Maybe my story starts in summer 2012, when I first heard about intermittent fasting on the BBC *Horizon* programme. Despite having a huge appetite, and a love of all things foodie, there was something so compelling about the science. From the day of my first fast, I sensed this might be the diet that would finally work for me, for good.

Or maybe my story starts in my teens, when I began

worrying about my weight – and I embarked on the first of many torturous cottage cheese and crispbread regimes that always ended in tears. Though I was also in my teens when I decided to go veggie – a decision that did at least offset some of the unhealthier aspects of my diet, because I experimented more with fresh produce, herbs and spices.

Or perhaps it was in my early forties, when the weight kept creeping on, and I started getting rattled by the health consequences of being heavy, rather than worrying about how I was going to look in my swimming costume (I still worried about that, to be honest). With both my parents suffering from type 2 diabetes, plus a strong family history of breast cancer, I knew I was at increased risk of both if I stayed overweight. I was an intelligent grown-up yet I couldn't seem to control my size.

So many things came together to make 5:2 a life-changer: the sense of freedom from the constant low-level deprivation and boredom that 24/7 calorie-counting causes. The focus and sharpness I enjoyed on a Fast Day – and the effect on my taste buds as I savoured the flavours of food so much more.

Losing 1–2 pounds a week was also the right pace for me: I didn't feel it aged me or led to saggy skin, as more rapid weight loss can.

Setting up a Facebook group (www.facebook.com/groups/the52diet) was originally just a way to get mutual support on this new approach to eating – but it soon became a brilliant resource as I decided to put what I'd learned into my first book on fasting, *The 5:2 Diet Book*. Then my publishers asked me if I had any recipes…

5:2 Veggie and Vegan is my fifth 5:2 book, and the one that most closely reflects how I live my life. I always fast once or twice a week (except on holiday) and though my weight might fluctuate by two or three pounds, as I approach my fifth Fastiversary, I am still two stone lighter, and a comfortable UK size 10–12. And my books have now been published in more than 15 languages.

The last five years have had their challenges and difficulties, but 5:2 is a keeper for me, something I can use as an anchor. On Mondays, I always look forward to the feelings of vitality and freedom it gives me.

I read all the new intermittent fasting research, and am particularly interested in how the gut microbiome influences our appetite and overall health: I'm changing what I eat – including even more fresh and fermented foods – to help all those friendly bacteria help me…

Our Facebook group now has over 55,000 members from all over the world. I'm still there very regularly, in between writing and recipe testing. It's a fantastic self-supporting community, with some dedicated volunteers who help advise the newcomers, and a wonderful and increasing set of fabulous stories. I love reading how people's lives have been changed: it really does feel as though we're all in it together.

Fast Day routine:

I never have breakfast but I do have a couple of black coffees in the morning. Then in summer, I'll typically have a salad for lunch with mozzarella cheese, homemade pâté or falafel, or roasted veg, and perhaps an egg dish for supper. In winter, it's soups or veggie curries all the way – my freezer is full of goodies, many developed for this book.

The other 5 days:
You can read all about those on page 305. But I don't ban anything from my diet.

The veggie life:
I can't imagine not being a veggie now, though I do cook fish and meat for my partner, Rich, and omnivorous friends. I don't like trying to change people's minds by arguing – I'd rather cook them great veggie food and prove how delicious meat-free eating is. And I'm so lucky living in Brighton, where indie food producers and restaurants are always coming up with new plant-based dishes and ideas. There's nowhere else I'd rather lead my veggie life.

Top tip:
Apart from all the advice in this book? Just give it a try. Every journey starts with a single step and we're all with you....

Last word:
I ♥ 5:2.

5:2 Know-how

YOUR GUIDE TO MAKING FAST DAY COOKING AND EATING A BREEZE

Developing recipes for all my 5:2 books has taught me so much about preparing and cooking food that is good for you *and* tastes great. In this know-how section I'm sharing my tips so that you can shop well, cook well and eat well – with the minimum of effort.

Fast Day shopping tips

Whether you're a veggie, vegan or omnivore, your shopping choices can make a real difference to how healthy you are – and how the environment, animals and human workers are treated by producers and companies. Both fasting and choosing more plant-based ingredients can save money on your bills – so you may be able to afford food with higher welfare standards.

Be label savvy

- **Read** the small print, front and back, and learn what the symbols mean. 'Traffic light' labels allow you to compare different foods, such as ready meals or snacks, to see which are high in sugars, salts and fats. And don't forget 'reduced-fat' is not the same as low-fat, or even as low-calorie.

- **Check serving sizes:** Manufacturers aren't always transparent about the calories their product contains: a serving can be half a pack, so you might eat far more salt or fat than you intended. Check nutrition per 100g as well as serving size to ensure you understand exactly what you're eating.

- **Look for E-numbers but don't automatically fear them:** All additives, natural or artificial, must have 'E-numbers' under European regulations; so E300 is Vitamin C, and E100 is curcumin, made from turmeric root. Even sugar has over a dozen different 'names', so you can see why cooking your own makes it clearer what you're eating.

- **What *doesn't* the packaging say?** If a label boasts a product is free from artificial colours, then check for preservatives: they're not automatically bad things, but Google is your friend if you want to discover what packaged food contains.

Where and what to buy

- **If you can, buy from specialists.** Buy from a farmers' market, local butcher, fishmonger or the grower at the farm door – you'll be able to ask more about how the food was produced.

- **Vegetable box schemes** are a great way of supporting local farmers and eating seasonally, especially if local shops are lacking variety.
- **Even veggie foods have an environmental impact** – avocados need a lot of water to grow well, so may contribute to water shortages, while rising quinoa prices mean farmers are selling their crops, rather than eating this healthy grain themselves: so they have a higher income but may end up buying more processed foods to eat. Higher prices can also lead to deforestation as land is cleared to grow expensive foods for import. There are no simple answers, but awareness of the issues, and where food comes from, is a first step.
- **Be packaging aware.** Look for shops where you can fill reusable containers with grains or other dry foods, which saves money as well as packaging.
- **Organic is more expensive but welfare standards will be higher, and pesticide/hormone/antibiotic use lower.** You can pick and choose organic depending on your concerns. The UK government publishes a report each year by the expert committee on Pesticide Residues in Food (PRiF) and the most up-to-date report, from July 2016, said no residues over the EU Maximum Residue Levels were found in apples, aubergines, bananas, broccoli, Brussels sprouts, celery, courgettes, lettuces, mangoes, pears, peas without pods, plantains, potatoes and radishes.

Ethical shopping tips

- Look out for logos on packaging for **welfare and agricultural schemes** that include checks on safety or welfare standards. For example, in the UK, logos include **Freedom Food** (meeting RSPCA welfare standards, which are higher than required by law) and the **Soil Association** (meeting organic rearing or growing standards).

- **Learn the language:** There's a world of difference between 'free-range', 'barn system' and 'enriched cages' when it comes to how laying hens live: most vegetarians would only find free-range acceptable.

- **The internet will help make sense of terms:** Sites like Compassion in World Farming (www.ciwf.org.uk) and Freedom Food (www.freedomfood.co.uk) offer advice on different agricultural products. The Good Shopping Guide (www.thegoodshoppingguide.com), Ethical Consumer (www.ethicalconsumer.org) and Shop ethical (www.ethical.org.au) offer advice, books or apps for use while you're shopping. Always look at the 'About us' sections of a site to see who is giving you the advice and how that is funded.

- **Speak up!** If you dislike a company's ethical or marketing plans, it's easier than ever to let them know, especially via social media like Facebook or Twitter. Ask questions, explain your concerns and **use your consumer power to change things for the better.**

There's much more detail on food issues, including GM, pesticides and hormone use, in my recipe book, *5:2 Good Food Kitchen*.

5:2 Know-how: your Fast Day store cupboard

If you put a bit of thought into stocking your kitchen, you'll always be able to whip up a tasty meal. Here are some Fast Day basics.

THE WORKTOP	
Oils	Olive for dressings and lower-temperature cooking; rapeseed or coconut for frying and roasting, sesame for Asian dishes
Vinegars	For dressings, drizzles and dips I use balsamic, white wine vinegar and rice vinegar most often, the last one for Japanese, Chinese and Korean dishes.
Eggs	I keep eggs on the worktop as they're a great standby if I've run out of other ideas for a quick meal! PS: They don't need to stay in the fridge, but keep them away from heat sources.
Fresh herbs, spices	See section below.

Garlic, tomatoes, unripe fruit, bananas	Garlic and tomatoes are so good for livening up dishes without adding too many calories – and tomatoes are so much more flavoursome if kept at room temperature than refrigerated. (PS: unripe fruit and especially avocados will ripen in the warm, especially if stored near bananas. Once ripened, pop in the fridge.)

THE CUPBOARD	
Storage	Grains, rice and pasta/noodles can all be attractive to insects, so store in airtight containers or sealed bags.
Nutritional yeast	'Nooch' is my new favourite ingredient: it's a vegan, non-live yeast that has a nutty, cheesy flavour and adds the extra 'umami' savoury flavour that food can sometimes lack. But it's so versatile, and because the B12-enriched version keeps your levels of this nutrient topped up, it's a particularly useful vegan source of the vitamin. Add it to soup, pasta and sauces.
Beans and pulses	Dried: there are so many kinds, but I keep red lentils, chickpeas and black beans as my legume staples. Tinned: more convenient as they're ready without cooking: chickpeas, black beans and cannellini are useful, as are kidney beans, which otherwise need a lot of cooking to remove toxins. Gram flour, made from chickpeas, is useful for pancakes and Indian dishes and is gluten-free and high in protein.
Grains	I rotate grains but usually have couscous, pearl barley, farro, freekeh.

'Pseudo-grains'	These are cooked as grains but are gluten-free and nutritious: they include buckwheat and quinoa.
Pasta	I always tend to eat whole-wheat pasta at home and keep a pack of whole-wheat spaghetti and one of pasta shapes, such as penne — choose gluten-free if you're coeliac, or intolerant. I like nutty spelt, but it's not gluten-free.
Corn	Cornmeal or polenta is good for soothing wintry dishes: popcorn kernels turn into a very quick snack.
Oats	Porridge oats are good for breakfast, baking, and adding texture to soups or bakes. If you're gluten intolerant or allergic, ensure the oats are packed away from other grains (usually marked on the packet if they are).
Dried vegetables	I keep porcini/wild, dried and shiitake mushrooms, plus dried chipotle peppers.
Tinned vegetables	Cheap and cheerful: I have sweetcorn and artichoke hearts in the cupboard.
Coconut milk	Coconut milk can enrich soups and curries, and is a great substitute for dairy, though high in fat. I buy whole-fat coconut milk but dilute it myself when I use it (cheaper than buying tins of reduced-fat coconut milk). The fat content varies according to manufacturer.
Tinned tomatoes	So useful: I keep tinned chopped and whole tomatoes, plus passata in vacuum packs, and a good tomato purée (all go in the fridge after opening).
Rice	A brown basmati rice is delicious and goes with most things. Try exotic rices such as black or red rice, too. On a Fast Day, just make sure you're using more veggies and a lower serving of grains/starches.

Nuts and seeds	Really healthy, though high in calories, so be very sparing on a Fast Day. Whole nuts: Brazils, almonds, cashews, pecans. Seeds: pumpkin, sunflower, pine kernels. Ground nuts and seeds: almonds, flaxseeds or a flaxseed mix for omega 3 essential fatty acid PS: I always keep nuts and seeds in the fridge **after opening** to help them last longer.
Pre-made items	Oatcakes: great for crunch, I like the rougher ones. Tortillas or flatbreads: useful for Mexican or Indian dishes and they have a longer shelflife than bread – can be frozen after opening. Bread – sourdough is tastier and lasts longer, plus it's better for the digestion than many faster fermented breads.
Soup and stock	I have a veggie bouillon powder for making soups: tinned soups can also be tasty and quick. Miso soup packs can also be very useful.
Sauces	Avoid sugary tomato ketchup on a Fast Day – look for veggie Worcestershire sauce, soy/wheat-free tamari, or hot pepper sauces to add flavour with fewer calories.
Pickles, olives, capers	Simple pickled veg can add flavour and crunch: try pickled onions, capers, sweet peppers, and also olives and jalapeño peppers in brine/water. Refrigerate after opening. Chutneys and sweet pickles do contain sugar but can add flavour to lower-calorie foods. Roast peppers, sun-dried tomatoes and other oil-preserved veg are higher in calories due to the oil, so drain as much off as you can by placing on kitchen roll before using.

THE FRIDGE	
Cheese: light halloumi or mozzarella, ricotta, light Greek-style salad cheese/ feta	I tend to avoid most low-fat foods because I'm wary of what manufacturers use to compensate for loss of flavour. But reduced-fat versions of halloumi, fresh mozzarella and feta are worth considering as they still taste pretty good. Ricotta is also naturally lower in fat. With full-fat hard cheese like mature Cheddar or Italian Grana Padano (which can be made with veggie rennet, unlike Parmesan), I generally prefer the 'real thing' – but use less of it!
Yogurt, milk and cream	This is very much about personal taste, but I choose coconut or dairy yogurt and cream: and dairy or almond milk for pouring/cooking: soya is another option, though it's also quite a common allergen. Calories in coconut/nut milk products vary very widely so do check the label. My fridge usually contains a large pot of full-fat Greek dairy yogurt, a lower-fat yogurt, and a half-fat crème fraiche. Goat's milk and yogurt is another option.
Tofu and tempeh	A firm tofu will keep for ages and is very handy for so many dishes. Tempeh is also worth trying.
Lemons, limes and other citrus fruit	Great for a clean, zesty flavour in so many dishes, and high in vitamin C. Keeps best in the fridge.
Quorn	Low-fat veggie (not vegan) ingredient made from a form of fungus and egg. The sausages or burgers are usually lower in calories than the breadcrumbed dishes.

Fruit	Berries, tropical fruits and ripe avocado that you don't want to ripen more.
Veg drawer	I keep spring onions, onions, mushrooms, red peppers, carrots and salad leaves (Little Gem are my favourite for ease of use) as my basics for salads and cooked dishes.

THE FREEZER	
Berries	Raspberries and blueberries freeze beautifully. Stir them into yogurt or use them in smoothies. You can also buy frozen berry mixes.
Leaf or chopped spinach	For when you don't want to prepare fresh leaf spinach: nutritious and super-fast.
Peas, broad beans, petit pois, edamame beans	Frozen just after picking, these hang on to their vitamins and are quick and easy to prepare. Also, higher in protein than many other green vegetables.
Prepared vegetables such as squash, roasted peppers, chopped onion or herb mixes	Perfect for speedy sides and suppers. I have had too many near-death experiences with cutting butternut squash to risk it when I am in a hurry; so I once bought ready-frozen and they're now my back-up plan for soups or stews where texture is less important (you can also cut squash more easily by roasting it whole before cutting into it). Frozen roasted peppers are also easy and tasty. And herb/onion mixes save time.

Herbs, spices and sauces

I could write an entire book about herbs, spices and sauces, but it can be daunting – and expensive – to buy loads of new ingredients.

Here are some of my must-haves, followed by some ideas for optional extras. Just pick your favourite cuisine or food region, and experiment... I keep my most-used spices on the counter, ready to use, in a masala dabba – an airtight circular tin with a transparent lid and seven pots inside plus a spoon (around £10 online). Generally, ground spices lose their flavour faster than whole, but you can grind your own from whole in a pestle and mortar.

HERBS, SPICES AND SAUCES	
Fresh herbs	I keep basil, mint and flat leaf parsley handy. They add so much flavour and colour to any savoury meal (and sweet ones, in the case of mint). I like the 'growing herbs' which are always fresh and appetising. If I buy herbs that are already cut, I wrap them in damp kitchen roll and store them in freezer bags or a plastic box in the fridge salad drawer. Woody herbs freeze well too.
Ground turmeric	Adds colour and flavour: very rich in beneficial compounds.
Ground cumin	Great for curries but also in Middle Eastern and South American cuisines.
Garam masala or curry powder (or spice paste)	Creates curries quickly, with minimal fuss.

Dried chilli flakes or powder	No need to chop: the quickest way to add heat.
Mixed dried herbs/ Italian herbs	People can be snobby about dried herbs, but if you replace every six months (once the aroma starts to fade), these are a good standby for grilled veg, pasta and tomato sauces.
Bay leaves	Inexpensive and keep for ages, ideal for soups, stews, etc.
Sea salt dish and black pepper grinder	Seasoning really makes a difference, especially to veggie food: if you're eating less processed food, your salt intake will be lower anyway.

HERBS AND SPICES BY CUISINE

For Indian dishes:	Mustard seeds, onion seeds (nigella), coriander seeds, cumin seeds, cardamom pods. Ground coriander. Curry pastes are also useful. Fresh coriander and mint leaves are a great topping or garnish and make a delicious fresh chutney (see page 196) or dip mixed with yogurt.
For east Asian dishes: (China, Japan, Korea and beyond)	Korean gochugaru chilli flakes are useful for kimchi (see below) and can be bought online. Soy and tamari sauce are both great for adding depth — tamari is gluten-free, while soy uses wheat in the manufacturing process. Hot green wasabi horseradish and pickled ginger are used with sushi but are also delicious and low-calorie with other dishes. Miso paste — start with a milder paste (generally the lighter ones) in a jar or vacuum pack. If you like them, try the darker, longer-fermented ones. Sesame seeds — black and white — good for garnishing many recipes.

| For south east Asian dishes: Thailand, Vietnam, (Indonesia and beyond) | Kaffir lime leaves are available dried, or sometimes fresh, and also add a citrus flavour to many Thai dishes. Warm spices such as nutmeg and cloves also add sweetness. Ready-made curry pastes are often more cost-effective than buying multiple ingredients, but do check the label as they very often contain shrimp or fish sauce.
Thai and Vietnamese dishes are rich in fresh herbs and flavours including coriander, basil, mint and lemongrass. Thai basil is particularly tasty, with a hint of aniseed.
Coconut oil and sesame oil both feature in stir-fries and curries.
Ketjap manis is a sweet soy sauce, quite high in calories, but delicious.
From tiny hot bird's eye chillies to fatter green or even orange varieties, chillies add so much to a dish, so do experiment with new ones when you see them, or seek them out in Asian grocers. You'll often find lemongrass stalks in the same stores, their aroma as delicious and fresh as the name. |
| For North African and Middle Eastern dishes | Imagine the scents of a covered market or spice bazaar: ground cumin, paprika, cinnamon and ground ginger. A single ras al hanout spice blend will give a good start. Pomegranate molasses and harissa hot sauce are both versatile and great in small amounts. The balance of sweet and sour is important in this region, so honey appears in savoury dishes too, along with ground or whole almonds. Lemons, oranges, fresh ginger and mint appear in cooking and hot/cold drinks and sherbets. |

For Mediterranean dishes	The freshness of Mediterranean cuisine relies on herbs and flavours that are fantastic fresh but can also work well preserved. They combine well together, too: capers, olives, garlic, lemons, fresh herbs such as basil, flat leaf parsley, sage, oregano and rosemary fill the kitchen with great scents. But dried woodier herbs also add lots of flavour.

Hands-on cooking tips

- Weigh your ingredients as you get used to Fast Day portion sizes. It doesn't take long – I keep small, cheap digital scales on the worktop and put a bowl or pan on top, adding ingredients as I go. It'll also help on non-fasting days. You don't need to weigh all the time to be more aware of what a portion size is, and which choices offer the most filling food for fewer calories.

- **Steam, poach or boil** vegetables and eggs – the easiest way to get good results without adding fat or calories.

- **Roast or fry using much less fat than you usually would** to get the taste and crispiness without the calories. It's easier if you use **non-stick frying pans and saucepans** which avoid burning or sticking.

- **Don't add more oil** if something sticks or burns, **use water, stock or lemon juice** to cool things down!

- **Grilling, or using a stove-top grill pan, is a great way to get flavour from vegetables,** while **dry-frying seeds, nuts and spices** before using in dishes helps release their aroma and flavour.

- **Seasoning makes a big difference to dishes:** freshly ground black pepper and a little sea salt, do pep up most foods. Though salt intake is something to watch, if you're eating fewer processed foods, especially cured meat and ready-meals, you can add a little to your dishes (as long as your doctor hasn't told you not to!).
- **Use vinegar, lemon juice or soy sauce to dress salads and cooked vegetables.** If you want to make more of a pudding out of your fruit, prepare it with sweet spices such as ground cinnamon or ginger, or a few drops of rosewater or concentrated natural vanilla/almond extracts, rather than sugar.

Batch cooking

There's nothing better than knowing you've got a freezer full of great dishes you've cooked yourself – except for maybe tucking into one! So many of the recipes in this book are suitable for freezing, so here are some simple guidelines.

- Ideally, use reusable freezer containers – I love the Lakeland Stack-a-boxes – hardwearing and space-saving, plus they come in small sizes for individual portions. You can also reuse pots with lids.
- Always label foods – even if you think you'll remember, there will always be something unidentifiable lurking at the back of the freezer. I also always add the calorie count and number of portions: ideal when you need

a great fast-friendly lunch or supper in a hurry!

- Add an extra layer of protection to strong-flavoured foods such as curries, so they don't taint other foods. A freezer bag wrapped around the box should be enough.
- I aim to use foods within 1–3 months of freezing: even if they're safe for longer, the flavours do deteriorate over time.

Soups	Wait until the soup has cooled down and pour into individual portion-sized containers. Don't add garnishes or yogurt before freezing. Either reheat from frozen in the microwave or defrost in the fridge.
Stews	Follow instructions for soups: if you have large chunks of veg or potato, reheat thoroughly so they're not frozen in the middle. For bakes, place in a metal container so you can reheat in the oven and preserve crunchy toppings.
Vegetables and pulses	You can freeze cooked vegetables, purées and pulses, such as cooked butternut squash or cooked chickpeas/beans. Don't refreeze veggies that have previously been frozen.
Patties/burgers	Open-freeze on a tray so they don't stick together, then layer between sheets of greaseproof paper or foil so you can cook one at a time. Either oven-cook, grill or fry in a little oil: ensure centres are fully cooked.

Fruit	Leftover berries such as raspberries, blueberries and blackberries can be frozen after washing. Strawberries don't freeze that well but can be used in smoothies, or frozen with peeled bananas to create an alternative version of the Bakewell ice cream on page 283.
Other leftovers	You can freeze hard cheese, butter, coconut milk, milk, cream, nuts and fresh herbs.

5:2 Kitchen kit: the tools of the trade

You don't need much kit to make brilliant Fast Day food, but there are a few good-value gadgets that will make your life *way* easier.

The basics

A box grater – for veggies, cheese, lemon zest, ginger and nutmeg

A medium **non-stick saucepan** with lid

A non-stick **small frying pan/omelette pan**

A sharp **kitchen knife**

A **stick blender** – the kind you use directly in a pan or bowl – to make soups, dressings and sauces fast and to a smooth consistency (you can get them for as little as £5)

A **pastry brush** – the silicone ones are easiest to clean – to apply oil or fat to vegetables, and marinades to tofu and other proteins

A **set of plastic measuring spoons** for ½ teaspoon, teaspoon, dessertspoon and tablespoon

The nice-to-haves

A **non-stick griddle pan** to cook vegetables, halloumi, or even fruits

Freezer containers – and labels so you don't end with a freezer full of unidentified stuff

A **julienne peeler** (or a spiraliser if you have lots of space) for courgetti

A **microwave** – for defrosting, reheating and steaming some vegetables

The luxury items

A '**Mexican elbow**' or citrus press: these are genius if you use lots of lemon and lime – the juice is forced out by an arm mechanism that is foolproof and fast.

A **food processor** – but only if you have space on the worktop or you won't use it!

A **pestle and mortar** – not expensive, and great for crushing nuts and seeds, and making sauces and spice blends

A **large non-stick stockpot** with a lid for batch-cooking soups and stews

A **large non-stick frying pan or wok** for stir-fries and larger portions of eggs, proteins, etc.

4

5:2

RESOURCES

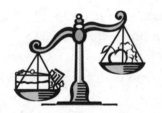

This part of the book contains tools and resources to help you plan your meals, understand your calorie needs and discover more about 5:2.

Recipes Listed by Calorie Count Per Serving:

The recipes are listed in the order they appear in the book, with two listings under different categories if there's a lower and higher-calorie option.

Under 100 calories

Cauli rice 🏵⊘🌾, 25

Purple chilli kimchi-kraut 🏵⊘🌾, 25

Lime pickled onions 🏵⊘🌾, 27

Coconut spinach 🏵⊘🌾, 35

Smacked cucumber salad with garlic and chilli 🏵⊘🌾, 35

Simple tomato sauce and variations 🏵⊘🌾, 38–54

Pistachio dukkah topping 🏵⊘🌾, 45

Pop-art coleslaw 🏵🌾, 52

Tropical fruit carpaccio with coconut and ginger cream 🏵⊘🌾, 54

Raspberry Bakewell ice cream 🏵⊘🌾, 56

Artichoke pâté with grilled red chicory 🏵⊘🌾, 58

Roast spiced chickpeas 🏵⊘🌾, 61

Strawberry and watermelon margarita salad 🏵⊘🌾, 68

Vietnamese spicy pho with fresh herbs and courgette noodles 🏵⊘🌾, 70

Super-green broccoli soup with an umami kick 🏵⊘🌾, 73/83

Rocket and ricotta frittata muffins 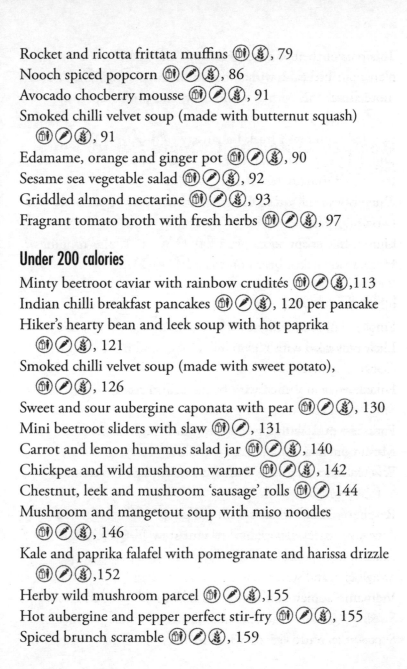, 79
Nooch spiced popcorn 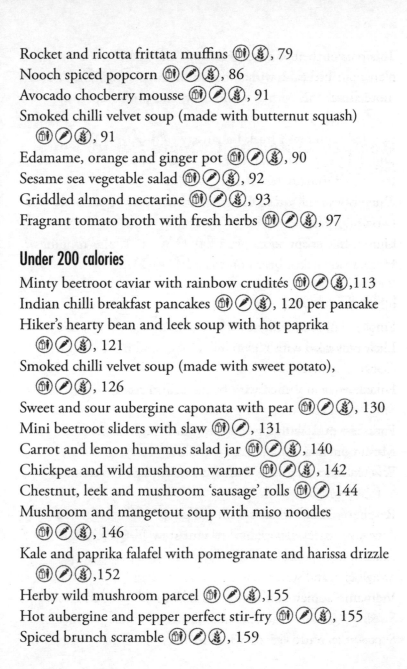, 86
Avocado chocberry mousse 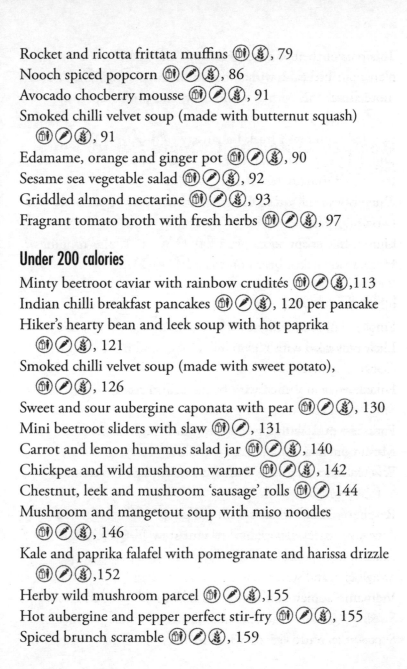, 91
Smoked chilli velvet soup (made with butternut squash) 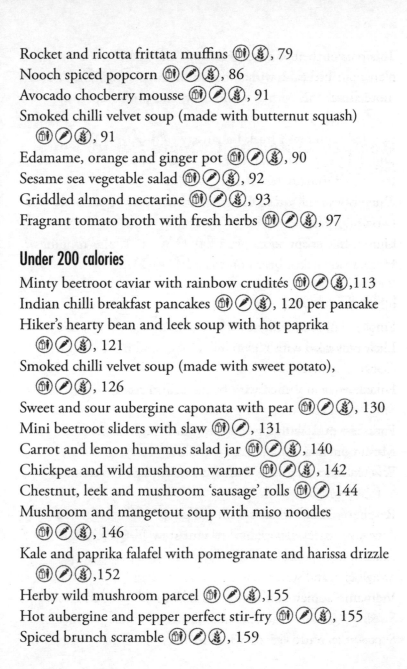, 91
Edamame, orange and ginger pot 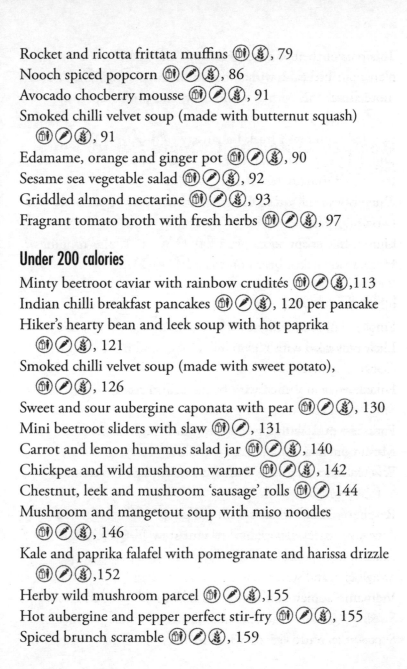, 90
Sesame sea vegetable salad 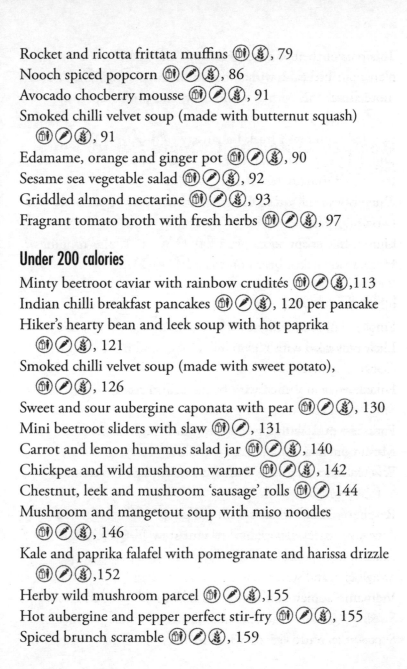, 92
Griddled almond nectarine 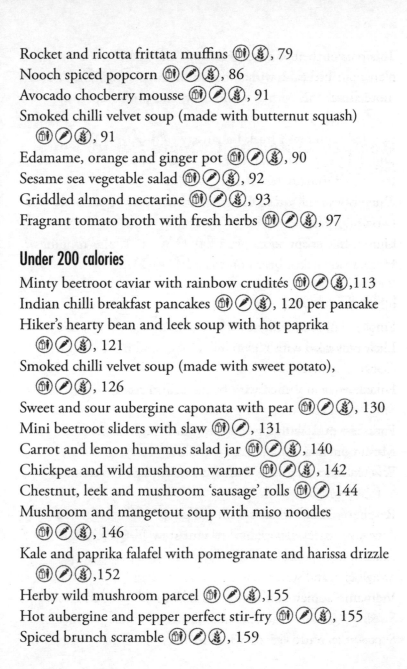, 93
Fragrant tomato broth with fresh herbs 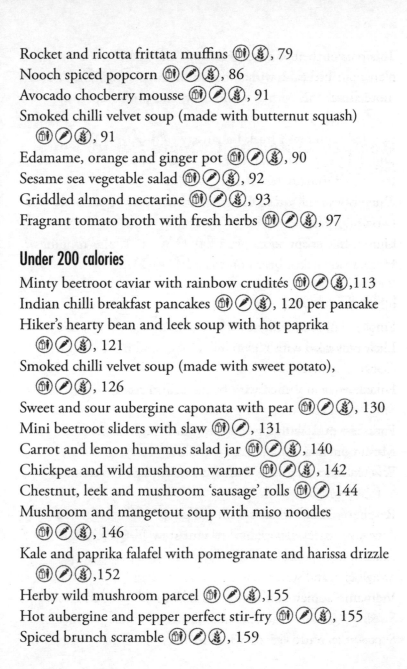, 97

Under 200 calories

Minty beetroot caviar with rainbow crudités 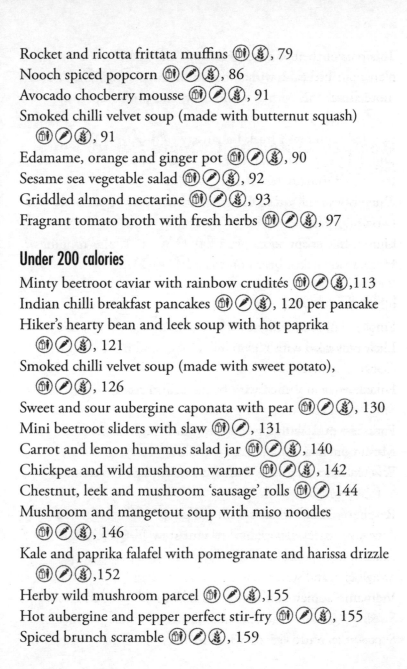,113
Indian chilli breakfast pancakes 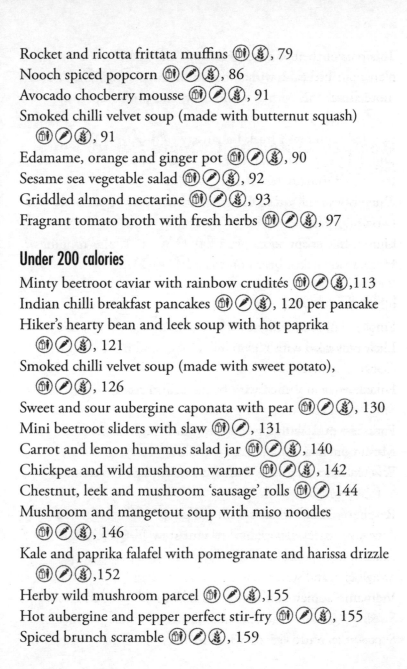, 120 per pancake
Hiker's hearty bean and leek soup with hot paprika 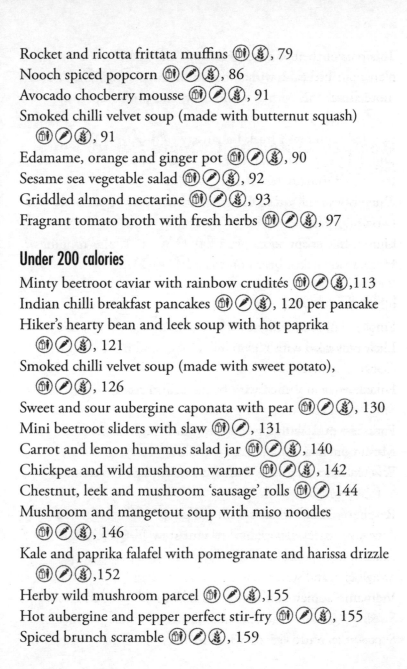, 121
Smoked chilli velvet soup (made with sweet potato), 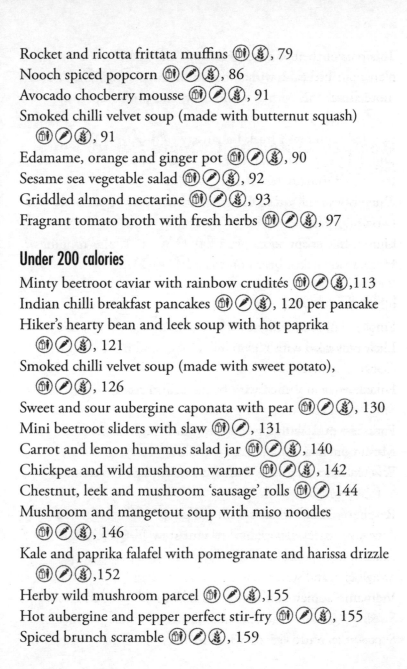, 126
Sweet and sour aubergine caponata with pear 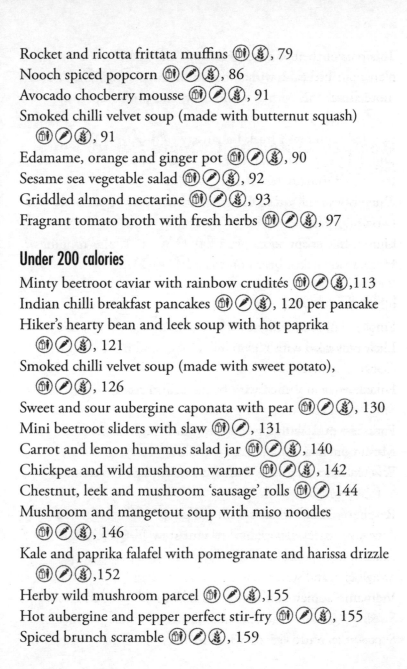, 130
Mini beetroot sliders with slaw 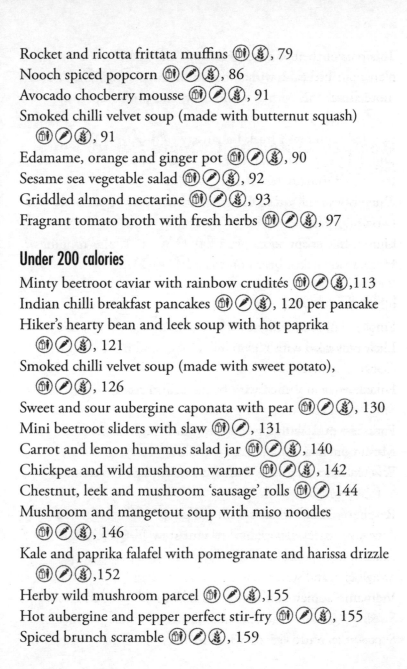, 131
Carrot and lemon hummus salad jar 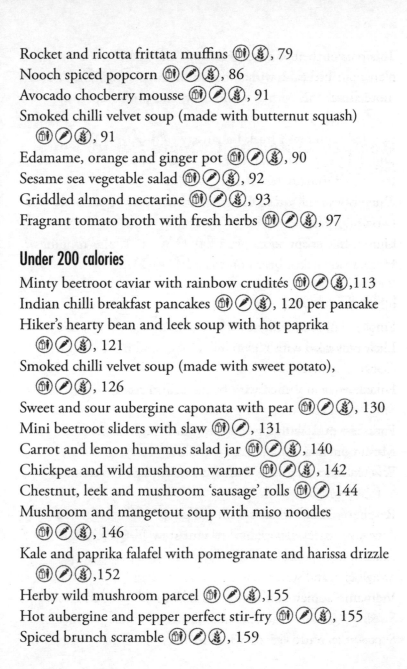, 140
Chickpea and wild mushroom warmer 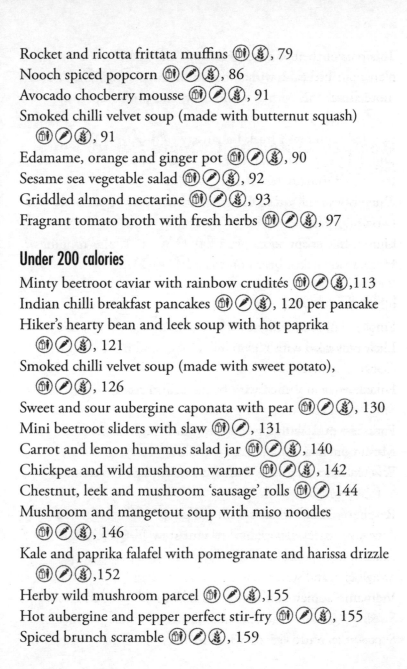, 142
Chestnut, leek and mushroom 'sausage' rolls 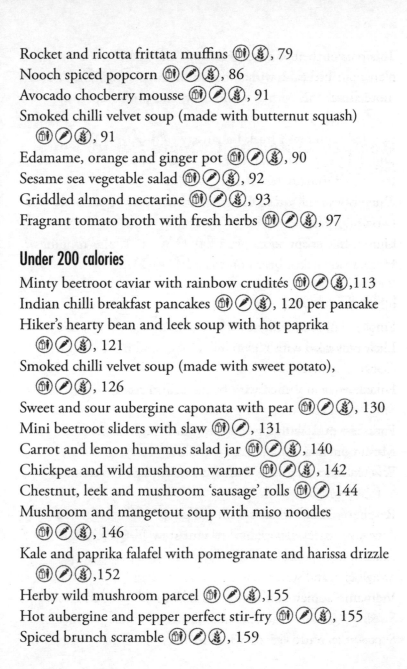 144
Mushroom and mangetout soup with miso noodles 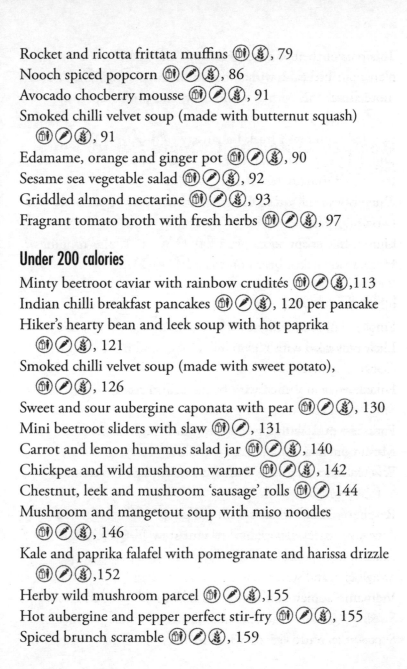, 146
Kale and paprika falafel with pomegranate and harissa drizzle ,152
Herby wild mushroom parcel ,155
Hot aubergine and pepper perfect stir-fry , 155
Spiced brunch scramble , 159

Super-savoury miso aubergine (V)(VG)(GF), 163

Korean grilled cauli with sweet chilli sauce (V)(VG)(GF), 165

Aussie smoothie with avocado, kiwi and pink grapefruit (V)(VG)(GF), 169

Roasted cauliflower steak Italian-style (V)(VG)(GF), 179

Onion bhaji lunchbox omelette (V)(GF), 179

Peach and tomato panzanella (V), 185

Open butternut squash lasagne with almond vegan pesto (V)(VG), 191

Gluten-free crispy socca pizza (V)(VG)(GF), 191, plus toppings

Homemade baked beans on toast (V)(VG)(GF), 195

Under 300 calories

Smoky soul food gumbo with vegan sausage (V)(VG), 200

Halloumi salad with melon, cucumber and mint (V)(GF), 203

Baked avocado stuffed with beans and smoked cheese (V)(GF), 209

Yorkshire puds with sage and mustard mushrooms (V), 211

Mushroom and chilli jam quesadilla (V)(GF), 213

BBQ kumara and beets with a crunchy pistachio dukkah topping (V)(VG)(GF), 215

Peacamole mint tostadas with red pepper (V)(VG)(GF), 218

Senegalese spicy squash and peanut stew (V)(VG)(GF), 220

Pea and herb pancakes with watercress and poached eggs (V)(GF), 222

Individual tomato and onion tarte tatin (V)(VG), 225

Sweet potato and black bean chilli with smoked paprika cream/avocado (V)(VG)(GF), 226

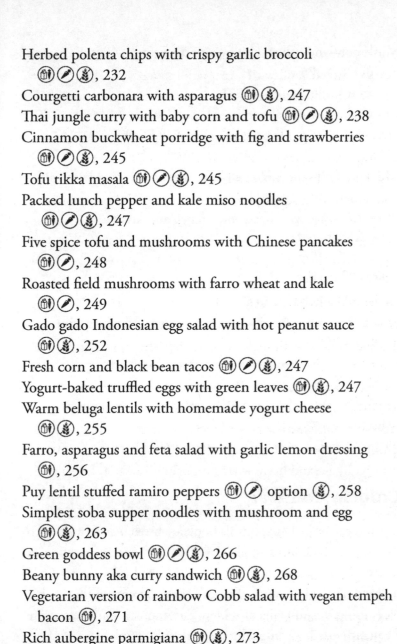

Mushroom and yellow chilli quinotto risotto with white wine ⓜ🥕🌾 275

Jerk tofu steaks ⓜ🥕🌾 276

Comforting lentil dal with fried spicy onions ⓜ🥕🌾, 280

Freekeh pilaf with olives, goat's cheese and herbs ⓜ🥕🌾, 280

Chickpea and pomegranate chaat street food salad with mint chutney ⓜ🥕🌾 286

Black rice salad with beetroot, orange and kefir ⓜ🥕🌾, 287

Under 400 calories

Paneer tikka masala ⓜ🌾, 301

One-pot spelt spaghetti with peas, thyme and white wine ⓜ🥕, 305

Javanese tempeh kebabs with sweet soy marinade ⓜ🥕🌾, 323

Vegan version of Rainbow Cobb salad with vegan tempeh bacon 🥕, 336

Hedgerow salad with blue cheese and blackberries 🥕, 361

Calorie Counter

Most of the ingredients in this book are listed below, with both calories per 100g/ml and also calories in an average portion or serving. The measurement is actually called kilocalories (kcal on food labels) but most of us call these calories so that's what we're using. In Australia and New Zealand, kilojoules are more frequently used – 1 kilocalorie equals 4 kilojoules.

Where a range of calorie counts is shown – for cheeses or tofu, for example, it reflects different brands and different production methods. Please keep an eye on labels to compare: you're unlikely to go far off course with white wine vinegar, for example, but with tofu varying from 65 to 185+ per 100g, it can affect your Fast Day intake.

For fats, I've **allowed 36 calories for 5g of butter and 41 for a teaspoon of oil**: though some oils and butters are a little higher, the amounts involved means the difference is very small. The juice of a small lemon/lime is averaged at 12, with 15 if you add zest.

The energy/calorie content of fresh produce depends on size but rather than weigh every carrot or onion, I've given averages. **Most vegetables are low in calories**, but watch out for the exceptions, like higher-fat avocado and starchy potato/sweetcorn. You may also find the calorie count for even basic produce such as carrots varies on packaging, because this changes depending on how new/old/starchy it is. I've adopted an average.

Some products, such as grated Italian cheese, nutritional yeast and desiccated coconut, **should be weighed on scales** as measuring spoons give inaccurate readings.

Herbs, spices, flavourings

I use dozens of different fresh and dried herbs, spices and natural flavourings in this book. Rather than measure each individual spice, I've made things simpler by allowing 5 calories for a small handful of fresh herbs, and 5 calories for a level teaspoon of dried ground or whole herbs and spices.

For some herbs and spices, the true calorie count *is* higher, but with such small quantities being used, it's not going to make a big difference to your intake. Salt does not contain calories and while pepper does, when we're just using it in small amounts to season a dish, it's not counted.

I've allowed 4 calories for a small garlic clove, small fresh chilli and a 5g/2cm piece of fresh ginger: again, there may be some variation depending on the size you use, but these ingredients won't derail your fast day.

Bay leaves, star anise, lemongrass and other flavourings that are removed from the dish before serving are not counted.

Food	Calories per 100g/ml	Average serving size	Calories per average portion
FATS			
Butter	730–750	1 teaspoon/5g	36–38
Oils, all, including coconut, olive and sesame	820–900	1 teaspoon/5g	41–45
DAIRY			
Blue cheese (e.g. Gorgonzola, Roquefort, Stilton)	325–410	25g	81–103
Brie (Light Brie – full-fat)	242–320	25g	61–80
Cheddar, full-fat mature	400	25g	100
Cheddar, reduced-fat	215–275	25g	54–69

Food	Calories per 100g/ml	Average serving size	Calories per average portion
Cow's milk, semi-skimmed	49	100ml	49
Crème fraiche, half-fat	175	1 level tablespoon	26
Emmental, reduced-fat	273	25g	68
Feta, full-fat	275–360	20g	55–72
Feta-style, light salad cheese	157–180	20g	31–36
Fromage frais, fat-free	50	1 level tablespoon	8
Goat's cheese	250–330	25g	63–83
Grana Padano (Italian Parmesan-style cheese)	385	10g	39
Halloumi, reduced-fat	230	50g	115
Lancashire cheese	370	25g	93
Light cream cheese	146–160	1 level tablespoon	22–24
Mozzarella, buffalo	270–290	½ a ball (62.5g)	169–181
Mozzarella, reduced-fat	160–175	½ a ball (62.5g)	100–109
Paneer (Indian cheese)	174–340	25g	44–75
Quark	69	1 level tablespoon	10
Ricotta	134	1 level tablespoon	20
Yogurt, natural, 4% fat	82	1 level tablespoon	12

Food	Calories per 100g/ml	Average serving size	Calories per average portion
DAIRY ALTERNATIVES			
Almond milk	13	100ml	13
Coconut, creamed	700	15ml	105
Coconut milk drink (diluted, in dairy cabinet)	20	100ml 'shot'	20
Coconut milk for cooking (varies widely according to dilution)	75–180	30ml	23–54
Coconut (non-dairy) yogurt	55–195	1 level tablespoon	8–29
Coconut water	18	100ml 'shot'	18
Greek strained yogurt, full-fat	95–130	1 level tablespoon	14–20
Greek/natural yogurt 0% fat	55–65	1 level tablespoon	8–10
Kefir, dairy	58	50ml	29
Kefir, coconut	35	50ml	18
Oat milk	35–42	100ml	35–42
Soya milk, unsweetened	20–35	100ml	20–35
Soya yogurt, unsweetened	40–60	1 level tablespoon	6–9
EGGS			
Egg, medium, UK size (58g)	131	1 egg	66
Egg, large, UK size (68g)	131	1 egg	78
Egg white	48	1 egg white	14

Food	Calories per 100g/ml	Average serving size	Calories per average portion
FLOURS, RICE AND GRAINS (grains all given as dry weight, before cooking)			
Baking powder	50–90	1 teaspoon	3–5
Barley, pearl, uncooked	352	40g	141
Basmati rice, brown	350	40g	140
Basmati rice, white	355	40g	142
Bulgur wheat	342	40g	137
Buckwheat	378	40g	151
Couscous	376	40g	150
Farro/emmer wheat	361	40g	144
Flour, white	360	1 teaspoon	18
Flour, wholemeal	330–355	1 teaspoon	17–18
Polenta	362	40g (baked slice or as a puree)	145
Porridge oats	355	40g	142
Rice flour	366	5g	18
Quinoa	365	40g	146
BREAD, PASTA AND NOODLES (pasta & noodles given as dry weight, before cooking)			
Bread, white sourdough	225–235	1 thin slice, 25g	56–59
Bread, rye	185–215	1 thin slice, around 50g	93–108

Food	Calories per 100g/ml	Average serving size	Calories per average portion
Bread wholemeal	220–250	1 thin 25g slice from small loaf	55–63
Filo pastry	290–355	1 sheet weighing 22g	64–78
Lasagne, dry	340–360	1 sheet weighing 17g	58–61
Noodles, egg (dry)	343–360	40g	137–144
Noodles, rice (dry)	350–360	40g	140–144
Noodles, soba, udon (wheat/buckwheat)	343–360	40g	137–144
Oatcake biscuits	440–450	1 biscuit	40–50
Pasta, white	340–360	40g	136–144
Pasta, whole-wheat	330–360	40g	132–144
Spelt spaghetti, whole-wheat	320	40g	128
Tortillas, corn or wheat	180–340	1 tortilla wrap (weight varies from 20g to 60g, so check packaging)	43–205

VEGETABLES AND SALADS (Given in whole vegetable or portions)

Food	Calories per 100g/ml	Average serving size	Calories per average portion
Artichoke hearts	30	½ tin, drained	36
Asparagus	27	4 spears	13
Aubergine	20	1 very small/baby (60g)	12
		1 medium (200g)	40

Food	Calories per 100g/ml	Average serving size	Calories per average portion
Avocado flesh	160	½ a baby avocado – 50g flesh ½ a medium avocado – 90g flesh	80 144
Baby sweetcorn	28	50g	14
Beansprouts	30	Handful 30g	9
Beetroot	42	½ vacuum pack, 125g	53
Broccoli	32	½ small head	32
Cabbage	26	75g shredded cabbage	20
Carrot	34	1 medium (100g)	34
Cauliflower	25	200g (florets only)	50
Celery	10	1 medium stalk (60g)	6
Chilli, hot	40	1 small (2–5g) 1 medium (20–25g)	1–2 8–10
Corn	90	1 cob 1 level tablespoon kernels	120 14
Courgette	20	1 small (170g)	34
Cucumber, with peel	14	½ small cucumber	14
Edamame beans	130	50g	65

Food	Calories per 100g/ml	Average serving size	Calories per average portion
Fennel	31	½ medium fennel	31
Garlic	110	1 clove	4
Green beans	30	50g	14
Kale	40	25g	10
Leeks, raw	30	1 medium (180g)	54
Lettuce	15	30g	5
Mushrooms, dried	250–275	5g	13–14
Mushrooms, fresh (button, chestnut, etc)	15–22	100g	15–22
Mushrooms, portobello	26	1 medium	18
Mushrooms, shiitake	25	50g	13
Okra, raw	40	50g	20
Onion, red or white	38	1 medium peeled	38
Pak choi, Chinese leaf	15–20	50g leaves	8–10
Peas, fresh and shelled	80	100g	80
Peas, frozen, petit pois/garden peas	60–80	30g	15–23
Peas, mangetout	32	50g	16
Peas, sugar snap	40	50g	20
Pepper	30	1 medium red pepper	30
Popping corn, kernels, raw	375	20g	75

Food	Calories per 100g/ml	Average serving size	Calories per average portion
Potato, white flesh, depending on type	70–90	1 small, 150g	105–135
Radish	13	3 medium	3
Rocket	24	Handful	2
Runner beans	23	50g	12
Sea vegetables/seaweed, dried	200–210	5g (rehydrates to 50g)	10
Shallots	24	1 x 10g shallot	2
Spinach	25	30g	8
Spring onion	32	1 small	2
Sprouted seeds and small beans, e.g. alfalfa, radish	30–40	20g	6–9
Squash, e.g. butternut	40	50g	20
Sweet potato, uncooked	90	1 small	90–120
Watercress	26	Handful	3
FRUIT			
Apple, with skin	47–50	1 medium dessert	60–95
Apricot, fresh	48	1	17
Apricots, dried	180	3 dried, ready-to-eat (about 15g)	27
Banana	105	1 small	89
Blackberries	40	50g	20

Food	Calories per 100g/ ml	Average serving size	Calories per average portion
Blueberries	57	50g	29
Cherries	60	10 cherries	50
Cranberries, dried	340	15g	51
Dates, medjool	287	30g	86
Dried mixed fruit	200–290	10g	20–29
Goji, dried	300	15g	45
Grapes	60	10 grapes	34
Kiwi fruit	55	1 kiwi fruit	42
Lemon, whole	29	juice of 1 lemon juice and zest of 1 lemon squeeze of lemon/a little zest	12 15 2
Lemon juice, bottled	24	1 level tablespoon	4
Lime	30	Juice of 1 lime Juice and zest of 1 lime	12 15
Mango	60	½ medium mango (mango weighing 200–300g total)	60–90
Orange, flesh only	37	1 orange	70
Papaya	39	½ medium (150g)	60
Passion fruit, flesh and seeds	36	1 passion fruit	17
Peach	35	1 medium	51

Food	Calories per 100g/ml	Average serving size	Calories per average portion
Pear	40	1 small, 120g	48
Pineapple	50	30g	14
Pomegranate seeds	100	1 level tablespoon (15g)	15
Raisins, seedless	300	1 level tablespoon	42
Raspberries	52	50g	26
Rhubarb, stewed, no sugar	7	1 level tablespoon	1.5
Strawberries	32	50g	16
Sultanas	300	1 level tablespoon	42
Tangerine/clementine	40	1 tangerine/clementine	40
Tomatoes	15–20	1 medium 1 cherry tomato	15–20 3–5
Tomatoes, chopped and tinned	20–25	400g tin	80–100
Watermelon	30	50g flesh	15
BEANS, PULSES, TOFU			
Beans, canned, drained, cooked (black beans, cannellini, chickpeas, kidney beans)	90–130	½ x 400g tin, chickpeas, drained, 120g	156
		½ x 400g tin, cannellini beans, drained, 120g	119
		½ x 400g tin black/turtle beans, drained, 120g	108

Food	Calories per 100g/ml	Average serving size	Calories per average portion
Beans, uncooked (black beans, cannellini, chickpeas, kidney beans)	320–350	25g	80–88
Puy lentils, cooked, vacuum packed	144	½ pack, 125g	180
Lentils, uncooked (beluga, puy, red and other dals)	300–340	25g	75–85
Tempeh	190	50g	95
Tofu (silken has lowest calories, flavoured and smoked the highest)	65–185	100g of most commonly stocked brands	115–120
NUTS, SEEDS, NUT BUTTERS			
Almonds, flaked, ground	575	15g	86
Almonds, whole, with skin	575	1 almond	7
Brazil nuts	680	1 nut	20–24
Cashew nuts	585	20g serving	117
Chestnuts, vacuum packed	160	15g	24
Coconut, dried, flaked	616	10g	62
Hazelnuts	668	15g	100
Peanuts, unsalted	564	15g	85
Peanut butter	595–650	15g	89–98
Pecans	698	15g	105
Pine nuts	695	15g	104

Food	Calories per 100g/ml	Average serving size	Calories per average portion
Pistachio	594	1 nut	6
Poppy seeds	556	1 teaspoon	28
Pumpkin seeds	582	1 teaspoon	29
Sesame seeds	634	1 teaspoon	32
Sunflower seeds	612	1 teaspoon	31
Tahini (sesame seed paste)	595	1 teaspoon	30
Walnuts	654	15g	98
STOCK			
Marigold bouillon powder	240–260	1 teaspoon	12–13
Vegetable stock, homemade (estimated)	3–10	500ml	15–50
SWEETENERS			
Agave nectar	300–340	1 teaspoon	15–17
Almond extract	Varies greatly, check label, up to 220	5ml (see packaging)	0–11
Apple juice	42	15ml	6
Cacao powder, raw	269	1 teaspoon	7
Cocoa powder, unsweetened	345	1 teaspoon	5

Food	Calories per 100g/ml	Average serving size	Calories per average portion
Honey	300–340	1 teaspoon	20
Maple syrup	260	5ml	1
Sugar, white/brown	395–400	1 teaspoon	15
Vanilla extract	Varies, check label, up to 288	1 teaspoon	0–15
70% dark chocolate	510–570	1 small square	30
SAUCES AND FLAVOURINGS			
Guideline for whole/ground spices (see introductory note)	100		5 per tsp; 0 per pinch
Most leafy fresh herbs	50		0 for a few leaves; 5 per handful/10g/ 1 level tablespoon, chopped
Branston pickle	109	1 level tablespoon	16
Capers	23	10g	2
Curry pastes	120–260	1 level tablespoon	18–39
Gherkins	25	20g	5
Ginger, fresh	80	2cm piece, peeled	4
Harissa hot sauce (varies very widely)	200–400	1 teaspoon	10–20
Ketchup	115	1 level tablespoon	17

Food	Calories per 100g/ml	Average serving size	Calories per average portion
Mango chutney	200–280	1 level tablespoon	30–42
Miso	165–200	1 level tablespoon	25–30
Nutritional yeast	343	5g	17
Olives, vacuum packed in brine	326	6 olives (15g)	49
Peppers, jalapeño in brine	27	Per pepper	6
Salsa	30–70	1 level tablespoon	5–11
Sriracha hot sauce	100	1 teaspoon	5
Soy sauce (lighter sauces are lower in cals)	50–120	1 teaspoon	3–6
Tamari sauce (lighter sauces are lower in cals)	55–195	1 teaspoon	3–10
Tomato chutney	130–160	1 level tablespoon	19.5–24
Tomato purée	75–100	1 level tablespoon	10–20
Tomatoes, sun-dried, not in oil	159	3–4 (15g)	24
Worcestershire sauce	113	1 teaspoon	5
VINEGARS AND MUSTARDS			
Balsamic vinegar	54–107	1 level tablespoon	5–20
Cider vinegar	18	1 level tablespoon	2
Distilled vinegar	16	1 level tablespoon	2
Mustard, Dijon	100–150	1 teaspoon	5–10
Mustard, English	175	1 teaspoon	9

Food	Calories per 100g/ml	Average serving size	Calories per average portion
Mustard, grain	154	1 teaspoon	8
Mustard powder	520	½ teaspoon	13
Rice vinegar	25–45	1 level tablespoon	3–5
Wine vinegar, red or white	22	1 level tablespoon	2–3
DRINKS			
Ale	25–47	½ pint	71–133
Apple juice	38–49	125ml	48–61
Black coffee	0–2	1 cup	0–2
Black tea	0	1 cup	0
Cava/champagne, dry	76	125ml	95
Gin/vodka/other spirits	222	25ml single measure	56
Lager	29–43	½ pint	82–122
Orange juice	36–43	125ml	45–54
Wine, red	68	125ml	85
Wine, dry white	66	125ml	83

Glossary

5:2, 6:1, 4:3 Different approaches to fasting or calorie restriction. The second number is usually the number of days you fast or limit your calories. **16:8** is a form of time-restricted eating (see page 303).

ADF Alternate Daily Fasting. Cutting down or eating nothing every other day.

B2b/
Back to Back Means having two Fast Days in succession, without a non-fasting day in between.

BMI Body Mass Index. Simple height to weight calculation used to gauge whether someone's weight may be putting his or her health at risk.

BMR Basal Metabolic Rate. This is what your body needs in calorie terms for basic survival, when not doing any activity other than basic functions.

Fast Fast usually means eating nothing (and, in some religions, not drinking anything either). However, 5:2 dieters often use it as shorthand for days when they eat limited amounts.

IF/ICR Intermittent Fasting/Intermittent Calorie Restriction. The latter is the more accurate name for the 5:2 approach.

Kcal	Kilocalorie is the accurate name for what most people call 'calories'.
TDEE	Total Daily Energy Expenditure. This is an estimate of the number of calories you'd need to fulfil your energy requirements for the day, which factors in your activity levels as well as age, height and weight.
WOE	Way of Eating – the phrase people often use in the 5:2 groups as an alternative to 'diet' to avoid the negative connotations that word can have for some of us.

Further reading/research links

If you're interested in finding out more about the topics in this book, especially the science of fasting, the body of studies and research about this subject is increasing all the time. Here are some great links and resources to help. You can also connect with others on the same journey to hear about their personal experiences.

The other 5:2 Books

My other four books about 5:2 are available as books and e-books from Orion Publishing.

The 5:2 Diet Book gives an overview of how to start, and the science, plus my very honest diary of my experiences.

The Ultimate 5:2 Recipe Book has lots more recipes and case studies, as well as lots of ideas for managing 5:2 on holiday, with the family and on a budget.

5:2 Good Food Kitchen has 80+ more recipes, meal plans, stories and also my *Making sense of...* sections to help explain controversial topics such as sugar, sweeteners and going without breakfast.

5:2 Your Life: Get happy, healthy and slim is an exciting six-week programme based on using 5:2 principles to become happier with relationships, work and even your sleep. This also has a six-week menu plan with new recipes.

I also recommend a well-written and great value e-book, written by one of the first members of our Facebook group, Linda Gruchy, *5:2 Fasting and Fitness: Easy Science in Layman's Terms*. And for a broader perspective on food, nutrition and the emerging science of the microbiome, *The Diet Myth* by Tim Spector makes for fascinating reading.

Help and support

You can't get much better than our Facebook group when it comes to day-to-day support, tips and encouragement: www.facebook.com/groups/the52diet. A visit to our website, www.the5-2dietbook.com, also has a great range of resources, including the Get Started section which includes more food photos, case studies and downloads to help you in your 5:2 journey.

For Fast Day calorie-checking, the myfitnesspal.com app allows you to scan barcodes to get calorie counts, and track your calorie consumption, exercise and weight loss. However, be aware that site users supply a lot of the data so they may not always be accurate.

BMI Chart

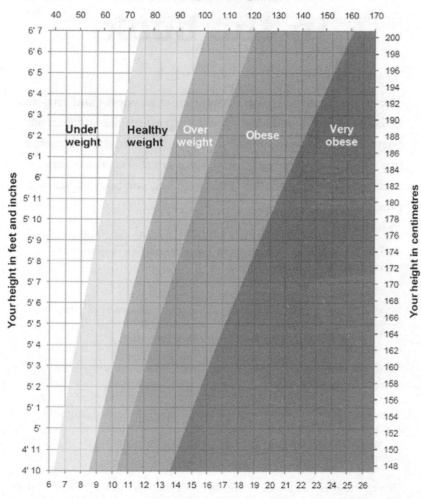

Your weight in kilograms

Your height in feet and inches

Your height in centimetres

Under weight

Healthy weight

Over weight

Obese

Very obese

Your weight in stones

References/ studies mentioned in the book

The following are abstracts or summaries of papers and reports available online, if you want to follow up on studies and research mentioned in the book. Please note you may need to pay a charge to access full reports, and the websites are all live at the time of writing (accessed 23/2/2017) but may become unavailable over time.

'The effect of intermittent energy and carbohydrate restriction v. daily energy restriction on weight loss and metabolic disease risk markers in overweight women', by Harvie M, 2014,
https://www.ncbi.nlm.nih.gov/pubmed/23591120

'Alternate-day versus daily energy restriction diets: which is more effective for weight loss? A systematic review and meta-analysis' by B. A. Alhamdan, 2016,
https://www.ncbi.nlm.nih.gov/pmc/articles/PMC5043510/

'WHO Obesity and Overweight Factsheet,' 2016, http://www.who.int/media-centre/factsheets/fs311/en/

'The effects of intermittent or continuous energy restriction on weight loss and metabolic disease risk markers: a randomised trial in young overweight women,' by Michelle N. Harvie, http://www.nature.com/ijo/journal/v35/n5/full/ijo2010171a.html

'Resting energy expenditure in short-term starvation is increased as a result of an increase in serum norepinephrine,' by Zauner C https://www.ncbi.nlm.nih.gov/pubmed/10837292

'Alternate-day versus daily energy restriction diets: which is more effective for weight loss? A systematic review and meta-analysis', by B. A. Alhamdan, 2016 https://www.ncbi.nlm.nih.gov/pmc/articles/PMC5043510/

'Caloric restriction and intermittent fasting: Two potential diets for successful brain aging' by Bronwen Martin et al', 2006 https://www.ncbi.nlm.nih.gov/pmc/articles/PMC2622429/

'Fasting: Molecular Mechanisms and Clinical Applications' by Valter D. Longo and Mark P. Mattson, 2014 https://www.ncbi.nlm.nih.gov/pmc/articles/PMC3946160/

'Meal frequency and timing in health and disease' by Mark P. Mattson et al, 2014 http://www.pnas.org/content/111/47/16647.full

'Role of therapeutic fasting in women's health: An overview' by Pradeep M. K. Nair, 2016 https://www.ncbi.nlm.nih.gov/pmc/articles/PMC4960941/

'Vegetarian, vegan diets and multiple health outcomes: a systematic review with meta-analysis of observational studies' by Dinu et al, 2016 https://www.ncbi.nlm.nih.gov/pubmed/26853923

'Vegetarian Dietary Patterns and Mortality in Adventist Health Study 2' by Michael J. Orlich et al, 2013 http://jamanetwork.com/journals/jamainternal-medicine/fullarticle/1710093

'Beyond Meatless, the Health Effects of Vegan Diets: Findings from the Adventist Cohorts' by Lap Tai Le & Joan Sabate, 2014 https://www.ncbi.nlm.nih.gov/pmc/articles/PMC4073139/

'Cross-sectional and longitudinal comparisons of metabolic profiles between vegetarian and non-vegetarian subjects: a matched cohort study' by Chiu YF et al, 2015 https://www.ncbi.nlm.nih.gov/pubmed/26355190

'Economical Healthy Diets: Including Lean Animal Protein Costs More Than Using Extra Virgin Olive Oil' by Mary M Flynn et al, 2015 http://agris.fao.org/agris-search/search.do?recordID=US201600087773

'Analysis and valuation of the health and climate change cobenefits of dietary change' by Marco Springmann et al, 2016 http://www.pnas.org/content/113/15/4146.abstract

'Low Protein Intake Is Associated with a Major Reduction in IGF-1, Cancer, and Overall Mortality in the 65 and Younger but Not Older Population' by Morgan E. Levine1 et al, 2014
http://www.cell.com/cell-metabolism/fulltext/S1550-4131%2814%2900062-X

'Sweetened beverage intake and risk of latent autoimmune diabetes in adults (LADA) and type 2 diabetes' by Josefin E Löfvenborget al, 2016
http://www.eje-online.org/content/175/6/605.full?sid=6eb5d176-c493-4834-8715-147b8da0dfad

'Antioxidants: In Depth', National Centre for Complementary and Integrative Health, 2013, https://nccih.nih.gov/health/antioxidants/introduction.htm

'Time-restricted feeding and risk of metabolic disease: a review of human and animal studies' by Jeff Rothschild et al, 2014 https://academic.oup.com/nutritionreviews/article/72/5/308/1933482/Time-restricted-feeding-and-risk-of-metabolic

Final 5:2 thank yous...

This book has been a labour of love for me: as someone who believes passionately in both 5:2 and veggie eating, it's been a pleasure to be able to bring those ideas together.

As always, the thank you starts with members of the Facebook group all around the world who've been sharing their highs, lows, photos and ideas since autumn 2012. I am so grateful for the help of our Facebook group admin team, past and present. The deadline for this book meant I wasn't around as much as I usually am, and you guys kept us all on an even keel: special thanks to Anne, Jane, Janine, Katharine, Linda, Nikki, Vicky and Wai.

Special thanks too to the lovely people who agreed to share their stories in this book: Heike, Liz, Jacky, Janice, Jo, Karen, Sanna and Suzanne.

Thanks to everyone at LAW but especially Araminta, Jennifer and Marina – and Peta for being there right at the start.

Many thanks to the great team at Orion for getting behind *5:2 Veggie and Vegan*, especially Amanda for her 5:2 cheerleading, and Emily for brainstorming, editing and the rest.

Thank you to Georgia May for making buckwheat make sense and to Helena Caldon for such brilliant attention to detail checking my recipes. Thanks also to dietician, Catherine Kidd, for her advice. Thank you to friends and neighbours for testing and tasting, and to Cally, Julie, Miranda, Rowan and Tam for their patience when I moaned about how many onions I'd had to chop.

As always, my love to Mum, Dad, Toni, Geri, Jenny and Rich. Your support means so much.

Finally, thanks to you for buying this book. If you've enjoyed the recipes, do get in touch to share your favourites via the 5-2dietbook.com – or leave a review for the book on Amazon so other people can find it too! And come and join us in the FB group, too, it's a great place to hang out: www.facebook.com/groups/the52diet.

Happy eating,
Kate

Index

Recipe Index

Farro, asparagus and feta salad with garlic lemon dressing 154
Five spice tofu and mushrooms with Chinese pancakes 252
Fragrant tomato broth with fresh herbs 96
Freekeh pilaf with courgettes, olives and fresh herbs 162
Fresh corn and black bean tacos 80
Fresh, fast Indian herb chutney 196

Gado gado Indonesian egg salad with hot peanut sauce 188
Gluten-free crispy socca pizza, with veggie and vegan toppings
  256
Green goddess bowl 156
Griddled almond nectarine 285

Halloumi salad with melon, cucumber and mint 150
Hedgerow salad with blue cheese and blackberries 166
Herbed polenta chips with crispy garlic broccoli 217
Herby wild mushroom parcel 66
Hiker's hearty bean and leek soup with hot paprika 98
Homemade baked beans on toast 70
Homemade veggie/vegan stock 108
Hot aubergine and pepper perfect stir-fry 178

Indian chilli breakfast pancakes 68
Individual tomato and onion tarte tatin 215

Javanese tempeh kebabs with sweet soy marinade 200
Jerk tofu steaks 191

Kale and paprika falafel with pomegranate and harissa drizzle 241
Korean grilled cauli with sweet chilli sauce 180

Mini beetroot sliders with slaw 259
Minty beetroot caviar with rainbow crudités 120
Mushroom and chilli jam quesadilla 130
Mushroom and mangetout soup with miso noodles 104
Mushroom and yellow chilli quinotto risotto with white wine 239

Nooch spiced popcorn 272

One-pot spelt spaghetti with peas, thyme and white wine 219
Onion bhaji lunchbox omelette 128
Open butternut squash lasagne with almond vegan pesto 236

Packed lunch pepper and kale miso noodles 126
Paneer/tofu tikka masala 197
Pea and herb pancakes with watercress and poached eggs 77
Peacamole mint tostadas with red peppers 132
Peach and tomato panzanella 148
Pistachio dukkah topping 249
Purple chilli kimchi-kraut 274
Puy-lentil stuffed Ramiro peppers 134

Rainbow cobb salad 158
Raspberry bakewell ice cream 283
Rich aubergine parmigiana 221
Roast spiced chickpeas 276
Roasted cauliflower steak Italian-style 223
Roasted field mushrooms with farro wheat and kale 250
Rocket and ricotta frittata muffins 118

Thai jungle curry with baby corn and tofu 186
Tropical fruit carpaccio with coconut and ginger ice cream 287

Vegan tempeh 'bacon' 160
Vietnamese spicy pho with fresh herbs and courgette noodles 91

Warm beluga lentils with homemade yogurt cheese 152

Yogurt-baked truffled eggs with green leaves 82
Yorkshire puds with sage and mustard mushrooms 209